Heart Failure

Advances in Prevention and Treatment

2020 Report

A Special Report
published by the editors
of Heart Advisor
in cooperation with
Cleveland Clinic

Cover image: © asiseeit | Getty Images

Heart Failure: Advances in Prevention and Treatment

Medical Editor: David O. Taylor, MD, Staff Cardiologist and Director, Heart Failure and Transplantation Fellowship, Heart & Vascular Institute, Cleveland Clinic

Update Author: Holly Strawbridge
Creative Director, Belvoir Media Group: Judi Crouse
Belvoir Editor: Kate Brophy
Production: Mary Francis McGavic

Publisher, Belvoir Media Group: Timothy H. Cole
Executive Editor, Book Division, Belvoir Media Group: Lynn Russo Whylly

ISBN 978-1-879620-78-0

To order additional copies of this report, or copies of *Stroke* or *Coronary Artery Disease*, or for customer service questions, please call 877-300-0253, go to www.Heart-Advisor.com/HealthSpecialReports, or write to Health Special Reports, 535 Connecticut Avenue, Norwalk, CT 06854-1713.

This publication is intended to provide readers with accurate and timely medical news and information. It is not intended to give personal medical advice, which should be obtained directly from a physician. We regret that we cannot respond to individual inquiries about personal health matters.

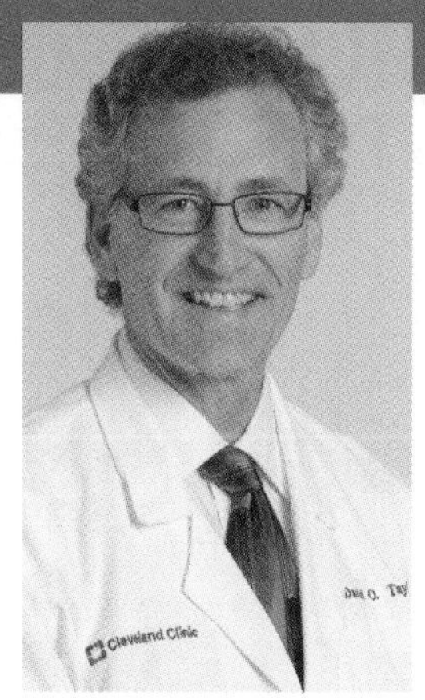

David O. Taylor, MD
Staff Cardiologist and Director, Heart Failure and Transplantation Fellowship, Heart & Vascular Institute, Cleveland Clinic

Heart failure is traditionally a frustrating problem, since treatment advances have been slow to come. But there's some good news in this regard. In 2018, we saw the advent of an exciting new class of drugs called angiotensin receptor/neprilysin inhibitors. These drugs dramatically reduce deaths and hospitalizations, while improving quality of life. In 2019, we added the first drugs ever approved for hypertrophic obstructive cardiomyopathy and transthyretin amyloid cardiomyopathy to our armamentarium.

Two excellent ventricular assist devices, the HeartMate 3 and the HeartWare, are being used with increasing frequency in people with advanced heart failure. Another device—the intra-aortic balloon pump—also has captured our attention with its ability to improve blood oxygen levels better than intravenous medications. In addition, we have learned that two pacemaker devices used in different ways also can help people with heart failure engage in their daily activities with more energy and less breathlessness.

Despite these advances, heart failure prevention remains the ultimate goal. The majority of heart failure cases are caused by heart attack and hypertension, both of which are preventable. That's why doing everything you can to lower your blood pressure, prevent a heart attack, and improve your health after developing heart failure is so important.

Use the information in this report to modify your lifestyle and reduce the risk of worsening heart failure. Understand why you must take certain drugs and keep taking them even when you begin to feel better. By arming yourself with knowledge about heart failure and its causes, symptoms, and treatment options, you may be able to maintain or regain the quality of life you desire.

Sincerely,

David O. Taylor MD

David O. Taylor, MD

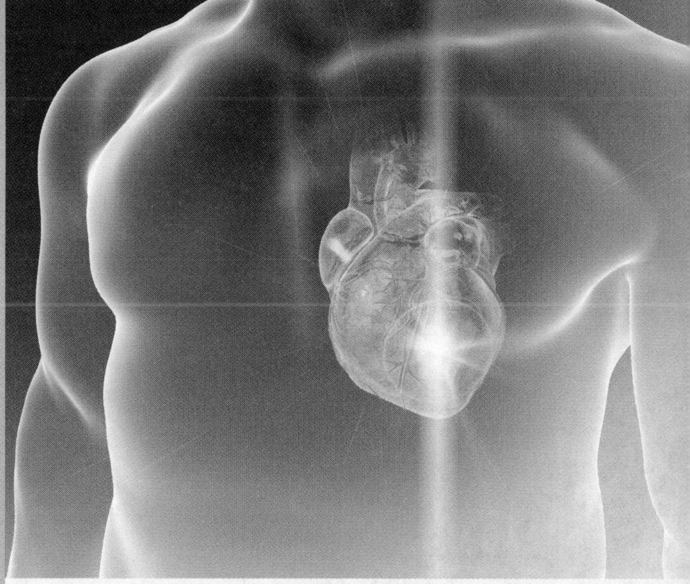

New Findings

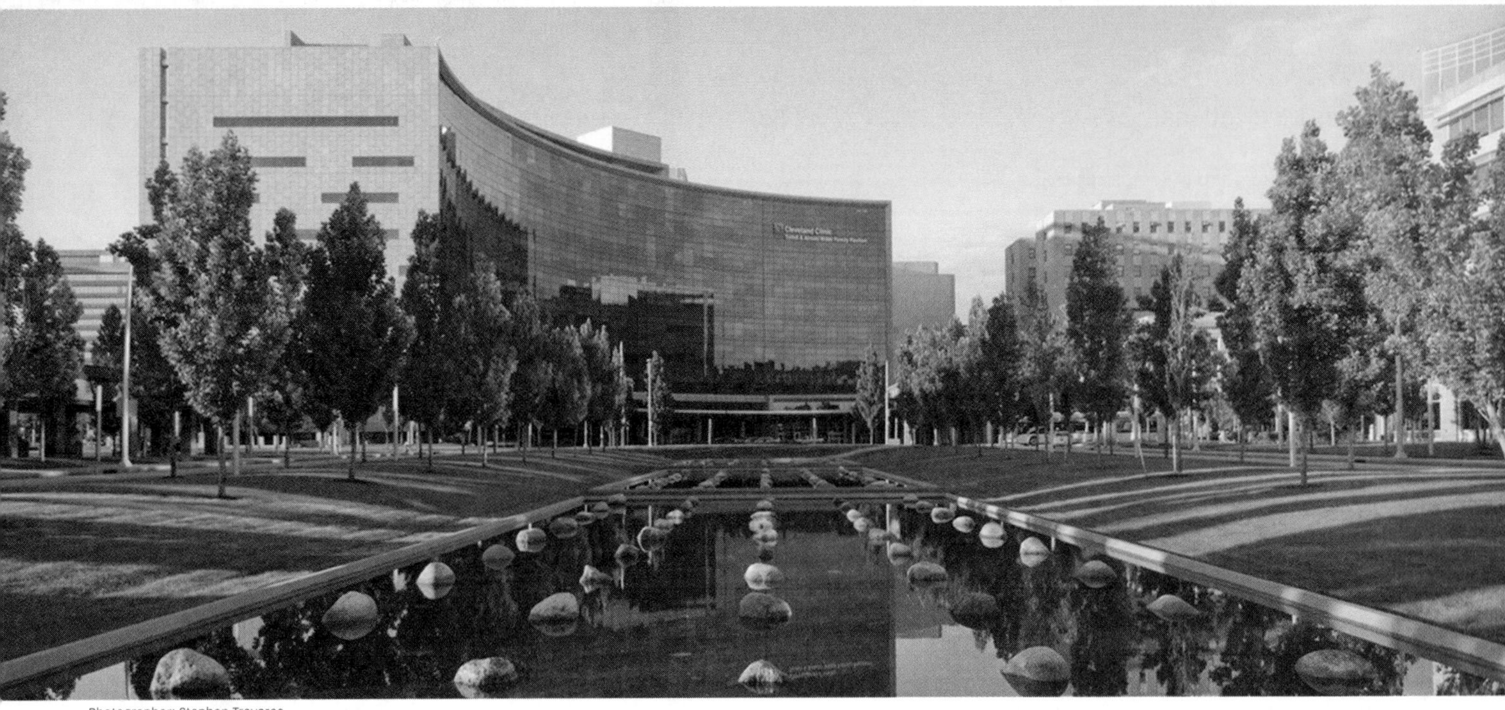

Cleveland Clinic's Sydell and Arnold Miller Family Heart & Vascular Institute has an international reputation for excellence, and treats heart failure patients from all over the world.

Cleveland Clinic's Sydell and Arnold Miller Family Heart & Vascular Institute is the largest and busiest heart program in America. It has been ranked No. 1 in the nation for cardiac care by *U.S. News & World Report* every year since 1994. Cleveland Clinic specialists have made breakthroughs that helped to define modern cardiac care—coronary angiography, coronary artery bypass, minimally invasive valve procedures, and refined robotic techniques, to name but a few. They continue to innovate for better outcomes and experience. With an international reputation for excellence, Cleveland Clinic welcomes patients from around the nation and throughout the world.

Cleveland Clinic services are provided through a unique model of medicine. Here are some of the factors that set it apart:

- **Every physician is a salaried employee.** All Cleveland Clinic physicians are salaried to ensure that patient care, not financial gain, remains their top priority. This practice eliminates incentives to perform unnecessary tests or procedures, and encourages physicians to consult with colleagues and spend the time necessary to practice excellent medicine.
- **Nurses and physicians collaborate closely on patient care.** Cleveland Clinic nurses are recognized and respected for the key role they play in patients' care, and are encouraged to speak up when they note a problem or have concerns.
- **Every patient death is documented and reviewed.** In an institution that accepts some of the sickest heart patients in the world, this practice creates a learning environment that helps keep mortality rates among the lowest in the nation.
- **Research is encouraged.** So much early research is performed at Cleveland Clinic that its physicians and nurses are able to identify promising technologies early and begin using them.
- **Innovation is valued.** Physicians are encouraged to think beyond usual boundaries to find better ways of treating cardiovascular problems.
- **Education is fully supported.** Cleveland Clinic pays for physicians to spend time elsewhere to learn new procedures and techniques.
- **Cleveland Clinic uses advanced health information technology,** including

electronic medical records (EMRs). EMRs enable physicians to spend more time with patients and less time doing paperwork, and make care safer by providing instant access to patients' records at all times. By using state-of-the-art technology-based systems that are true medical tools, Cleveland Clinic is able to meet its physicians' needs and better serve patients.

Facilities for State-of-the-Art Care

The Sydell and Arnold Miller Family Pavilion—a 1 million-square-foot, state-of-the-art center that opened in 2008—is dedicated exclusively to heart and vascular care. The pavilion includes such features as robotic surgery suites; facilities for more than 6,000 diagnostic catheterizations and 1,800 interventional procedures a year; operating rooms for 4,500 cardiac and 3,000 valve surgeries a year; electrophysiology labs for 1,600 ablations, 1,600 device implantations, and lead extractions a year; 10 heart failure intensive care beds; 24 coronary intensive care beds; 76 cardiac and vascular surgery beds; and 283 private patient rooms. Cutting-edge cardiac radiology and nuclear medicine services are provided on site, and the center includes a 21-bed kidney dialysis suite, as well as a rooftop helipad to receive critically ill or injured patients.

The Miller Family Heart & Vascular Institute at Cleveland Clinic, the country's largest cardiovascular practice, employs more than 300 physicians within the Robert and Suzanne Tomsich Department of Cardiovascular Medicine, the Department of Thoracic and Cardiothoracic Surgery, and the Department of Vascular Surgery.

Cleveland Clinic is a recipient of the American Heart Association's Get With the Guidelines® Gold Award for greatest success in improving the quality of care for people with heart failure. By following these guidelines, Cleveland Clinic is able to improve the quality of care for heart failure patients and help prevent future hospitalizations from occurring.

About the George M. and Linda H. Kaufman Center for Heart Failure

In 1997, Cleveland Clinic established the George M. and Linda H. Kaufman Center for Heart Failure with a multimillion-dollar gift from the Kaufmans and additional funds from other philanthropic sources and grants. The center is a collaborative effort by some of the world's leading specialists in heart failure to advance the diagnosis and treatment of this pervasive medical problem.

The center facilitates Cleveland Clinic's participation in clinical trials of investigational treatments, as well as innovative use of standard therapies for heart failure. Close collaboration among cardiologists, cardiac surgeons, and research scientists provides cutting-edge technology to patients.

About Cleveland Clinic: A History of Innovation

Discoveries and Advances

- Breakthroughs in understanding high blood pressure and its links to heart disease
- Pioneering open-heart surgery on a stopped heart
- Discovery of the enzyme angiotensin and its role in high blood pressure
- Development of implantable artificial hearts
- Discovery of coronary angiography
- Discovery of the first gene associated with familial heart attacks
- Creation of a test for myeloperoxidase, a biomarker for heart attack

Innovations and Firsts

- First coronary artery bypass surgery
- First dedicated cardiothoracic anesthesiology department
- First heart transplant in Ohio
- First heart/double-lung transplant in Ohio
- First heart-liver transplant in Ohio
- First minimally invasive mitral valve operation in the world
- First computerized database for cardiovascular diagnosis and treatment
- Invention of a clip device to exclude the left atrial appendage and prevent stroke in patients with atrial fibrillation
- Development of tissue-lined stent to treat peripheral vascular disease
- Development of implantable artificial hearts
- Development of an annuloplasty ring for valve repair
- Invention of closure device for repairing septal defects

Therapies and Procedures

- Pioneering work with arterial bypass grafts in cardiac surgery, which has increased survival rates
- Development of blood-conservation techniques to eliminate the need for transfusion in many patients
- Development of new valve-repair techniques
- Introduction of intravenous thrombolytic (clot-busting) therapy for heart attacks
- Use of intravascular ultrasound to visualize plaque in artery walls
- Pioneering of surgical treatment for atrial fibrillation
- Development of a debris catcher to improve the safety of carotid stenting

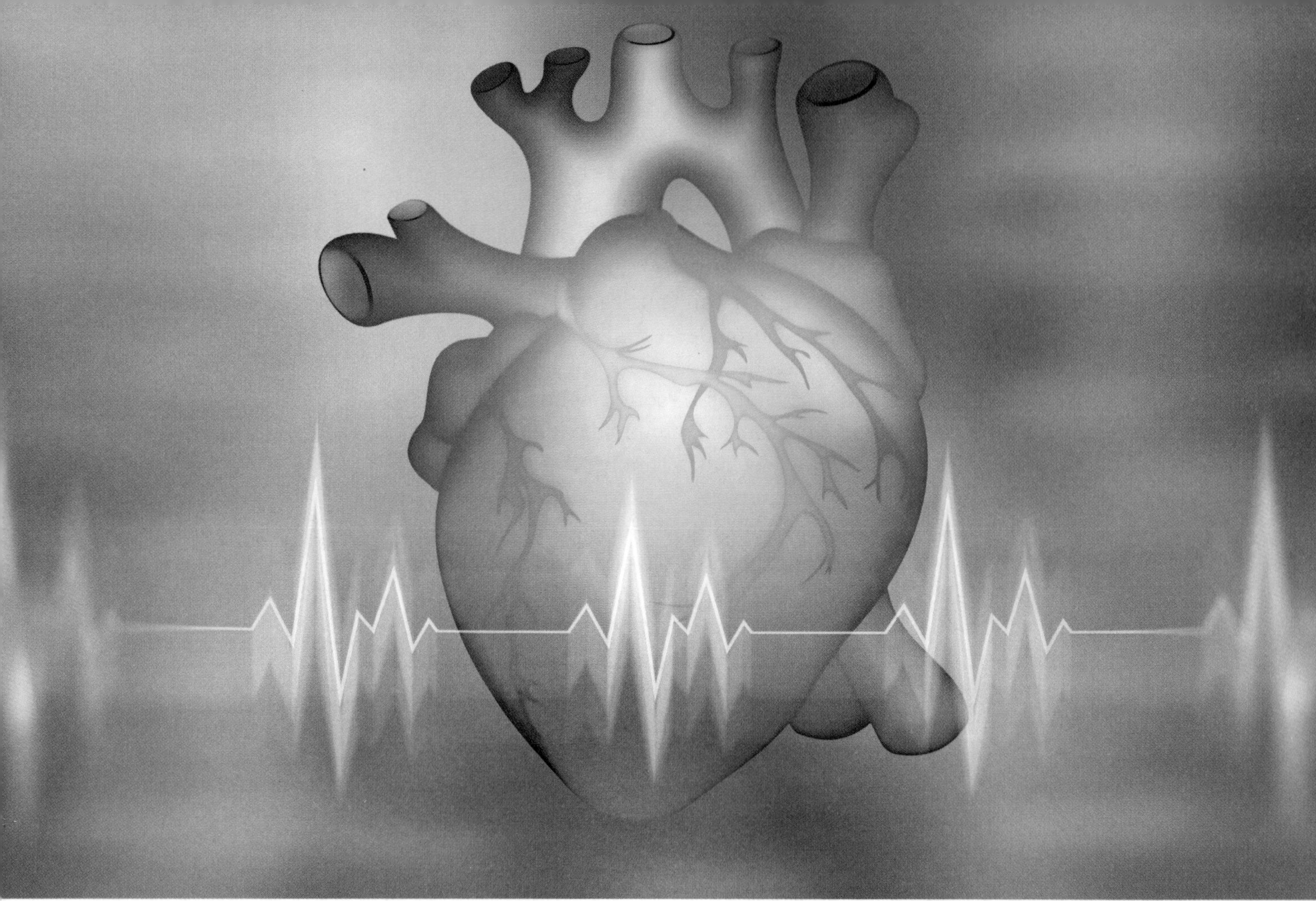

© Siarhei Yurchanka | Dreamstime

Medical advances have ensured that more people are surviving heart attacks—but this has resulted in an increase in heart failure incidence.

1 "You Have Heart Failure"

There's no question that heart failure is a serious condition. It's also very common. One in every five U.S. adults will develop heart failure in their lifetime. According to the latest American Heart Association statistics, heart failure affects an estimated 6.2 million people age 20 and older in this country, and it's on the rise—by the year 2030, the number of people affected by the condition is expected to exceed 8 million and may be as high as 10 million. That's an astounding figure for a condition that is primarily preventable.

The high prevalence of heart failure is largely due to the fact that more people are surviving heart attacks and living with damaged hearts. Since coronary artery disease and heart attacks are most likely to occur in older people, and the link between these diseases and heart failure has been well established, it follows that the incidence of heart failure increases with age.

The High Cost of Heart Failure

Heart failure is an expensive health problem, costing the United States nearly $31 billion a year. If the number of Americans with heart failure rises as expected, it may cost as much as $70 billion by 2030 to treat the condition.

The high cost of heart failure can be attributed to the need for ongoing, often expensive, medical care. When people with heart failure experience a sudden increase in symptoms such as difficulty breathing, they often need to be hospitalized. This is known as acute decompensated heart failure, and it is a sign the condition is worsening. In 2015, there were 2,671,000 physician office visits for heart failure, and 481,000 emergency department visits. One study found that 83 percent of people with heart failure were hospitalized at least once, and 43 percent up to four times.

Far-Reaching Effects on Quality of Life

A serious issue that affects people with heart failure is declining quality of life. Unfortunately, the condition can be disabling. About half of heart failure patients require home care or nursing home care. Simple activities, such as walking across a room or grocery shopping, become challenging.

Proactive Management Is Vital

Keeping people with heart failure functioning as well as possible and out of the hospital is a time-consuming job. Heart failure is such a complex problem that optimal care is best provided by a team of physicians who work collaboratively with patients and their caregivers to achieve shared goals.

While new treatments and innovative approaches to heart failure management can enhance quality of life for people with the condition, 78,356 U.S. adults died from heart failure in 2016. That figure is 28 percent higher than it was in 2005. The likelihood of dying after heart-failure hospitalization is more than 10 percent at one year and 42 percent at three years. This makes it imperative to do everything possible to protect your health if

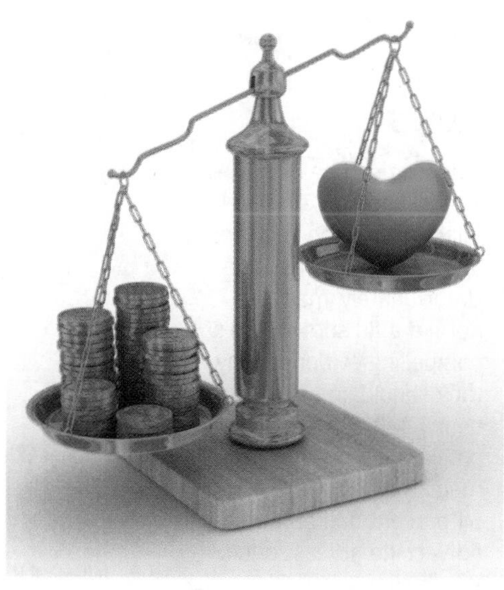

Heart failure costs the United States nearly $31 billion each year, and this number is expected to rise.

Team-Based Care for Heart Failure Works Best

Heart failure is such a complex problem that optimal care is best provided by a team of physicians who work collaboratively with patients and their caregivers to achieve shared goals. This was the conclusion of experts on the American College of Cardiology's Heart Failure Pathway Writing Committee, who arrived at a consensus on how physicians should make clinical treatment decisions based on best evidence garnered from clinical trials.

Treating heart failure in general, and heart failure with reduced ejection fraction (HFrEF) in particular, is complex because of the breadth and depth of treatments available. These include multiple medications, sophisticated devices, surgery, and lifestyle changes. Understanding when and how to add, switch, and titrate all medications to reach maximally tolerated doses and, ideally, target doses is a challenge for cardiologists. Many patients with HFrEF require additional care from an electrophysiologist if a device must be implanted, monitored, or adjusted.

Additionally, heart failure patients commonly have other heart and non-heart medical problems. In fact, more than 50 percent of Medicare patients with heart failure have four or more non-cardiovascular issues, and 25 percent have six or more. This raises the risk of poorly coordinated care, miscommunications, potential medication interactions, drug-disease interactions, and other problems that interfere with achieving optimal outcomes.

This is why team-based care is considered the most effective approach to managing complex heart failure. Clinical trials have shown that heart failure patients cared for by a team have better quality of life, fewer hospitalizations, shorter lengths of stay when they are hospitalized, and fewer deaths. These outcomes are achieved through greater adherence to guideline-directed medical therapy, effective doses of the right drugs, and earlier recognition of the signs and symptoms of heart failure.

By definition, a team is two or more caregivers. The size of the team is not as important as the individual caregivers' skills. These skills should include proficiency in monitoring for the progression and exacerbation of heart failure, care coordination, treatment prescription and monitoring, and education for patients and their caregivers.

NEW FINDING

Get a Flu Shot Every Year

Influenza can be deadly, and all people with heart failure should be vaccinated against the flu once a year. Unfortunately, many do not get a flu shot. There's compelling evidence why they should. In a study of nearly 135,000 heart failure patients followed for a median of 3.7 years, 16 to 54 percent had received the flu vaccine at least once. Vaccination reduced the risk of death from cardiovascular disease, as well as all causes, by 18 percent. Being vaccinated earlier in the fall offered greater protection against death, as did being vaccinated every year.

Circulation, Dec. 10, 2018

you have heart failure (see "Get a Flu Shot—Every Year"). The good news is that new medications and innovative mechanical pumps that boost the heart are helping more people with heart failure live longer and better. It is estimated that nearly 68,000 deaths a year could be prevented if all heart failure patients took advantage of all of the treatments recommended in treatment guidelines.

Positive Developments

If you have heart failure, you would benefit from taking a proactive role in improving your overall health. Eliminating risk factors, improving your diet, and starting an exercise program can go a long way toward improving your quality of life and possibly prolonging it. Learn everything you can about heart failure, because knowledge is power.

Equipped with information about the latest heart failure treatments, you can become a full partner with your physician in managing your care. Nevertheless, the outcome of heart failure for any individual is hard to predict. Some patients remain reasonably stable for years on standard medications. Others slowly slide downhill, despite aggressive treatment with advanced medications and mechanical therapies.

Your physician's goal may be to help you live longer. You may not share that goal if your medications produce intolerable side effects, or you are distressed at the idea of needing a mechanical device or heart transplant. Be sure you have all the necessary information to make a decision. Have an honest conversation with your cardiologist. Ask what lies ahead for you, and what your treatment options are. If you aren't satisfied with the answers you receive, seek a second opinion. You are much more likely to remain optimistic if you and your doctor work together toward a shared goal.

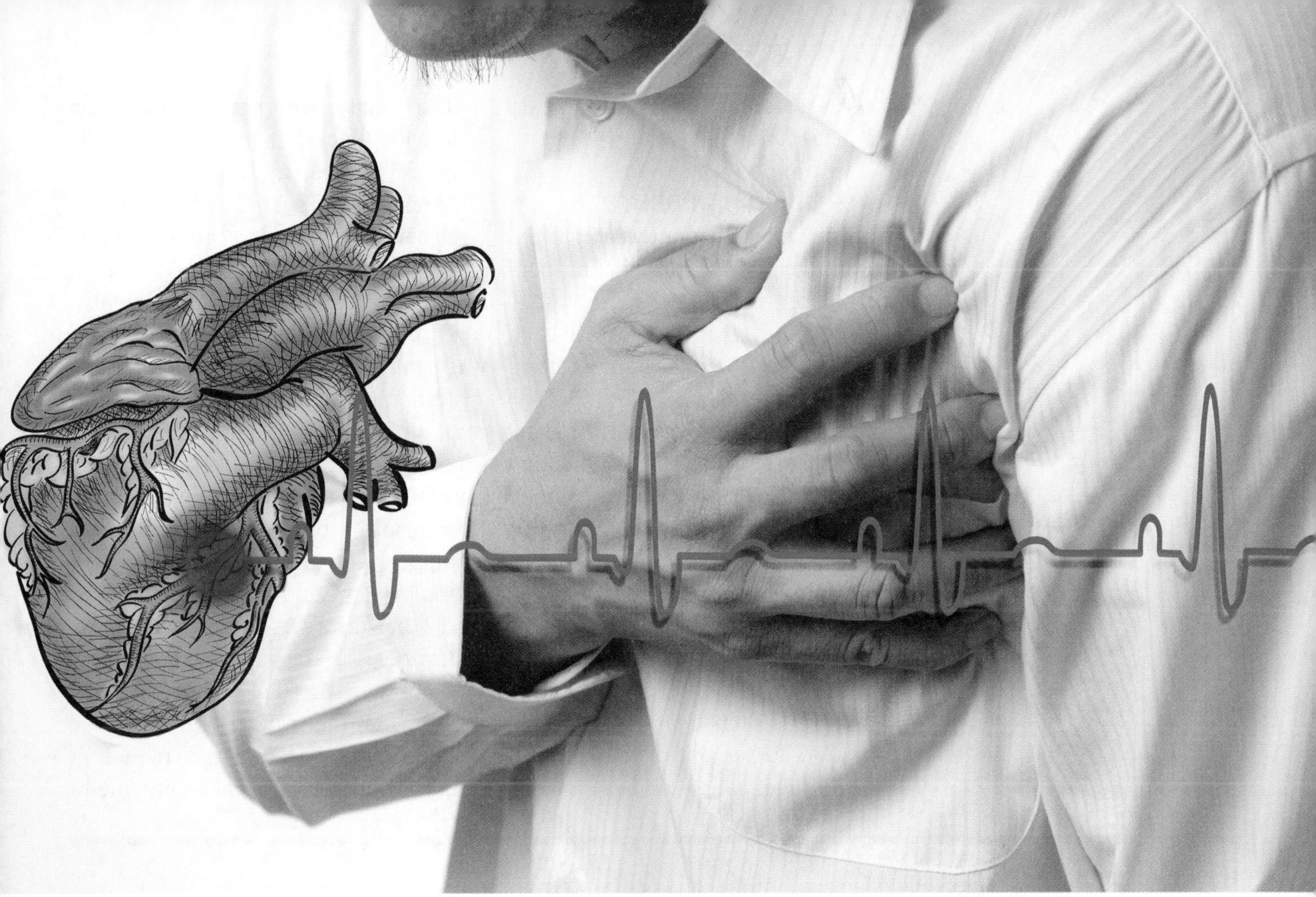

© Redbaron | Dreamstime

A heart attack is one of the most common causes of heart failure.

2 What Is Heart Failure?

Heart failure is a collection of symptoms and physical problems brought on by injury to, or weakness of, the heart. In heart failure, the heart is unable to pump enough blood to meet the body's needs.

Heart failure occurs gradually, producing symptoms—such as fatigue, shortness of breath, and fluid retention—that worsen over time. Although heart failure often is called "congestive heart failure," congestion in the lungs is not always present. For that reason, the condition is now simply called "heart failure." But even the term "failure" can be misleading, since today's treatments put some patients into remission.

How the Heart Works

The heart is essentially a pump made of muscle. Its strong, muscular walls contract and relax in a coordinated fashion to pump blood out to the body at a normal rate of five or six liters per minute at rest. The body's vital organs require this oxygen-rich blood to function.

The heart has four chambers: two upper chambers, called atria, and two lower chambers, known as ventricles. Valves strategically placed between these chambers open and close at the right moments to direct blood flow through the heart and out to the body without allowing it to back up. The atria pump blood into the ventricles, and the ventricles pump blood out into the lungs and body.

The heart must squeeze forcefully to pump blood to all parts of the body, but it also must relax between beats to fill properly with blood. If either part of this intricate system is damaged or weakened, heart failure can result.

Types of Heart Failure

Heart function is frequently categorized according to the left ventricular ejection fraction, which is the percentage of blood the heart pumps out with each contraction. A normal ejection fraction is 55 to 65 percent.

There are two types of heart failure:

- **Heart failure with reduced ejection fraction (HFrEF),** also called systolic heart failure. HFrEF occurs when the left ventricle becomes large and contracts so weakly that it cannot expel blood efficiently to the body. People with this condition have an ejection fraction of 10 to 40 percent. This means their heart only pumps out 10 to 40 percent of the blood in the ventricles with each beat.
- **Heart failure with preserved ejection fraction (HFpEF),** also called diastolic heart failure. In HFpEF, pumping strength is preserved, but the ventricles become stiff and cannot expand properly to fill with blood. Therefore, the heart cannot pump as efficiently.

Although both forms of heart failure can coexist, most patients have one type or the other. HFrEF is more common in men, and HFpEF is more common in women. This is likely due to the fact that men tend to have heart attacks that result in damage to the pumping chambers, and women tend to have high blood pressure, chronic kidney disease, and other disorders that can lead to a stiffer heart.

Women with HFpEF generally live longer than men with HFrEF. However, they tend to be hospitalized frequently, and have limited physical ability due to

How the Normal Heart Works

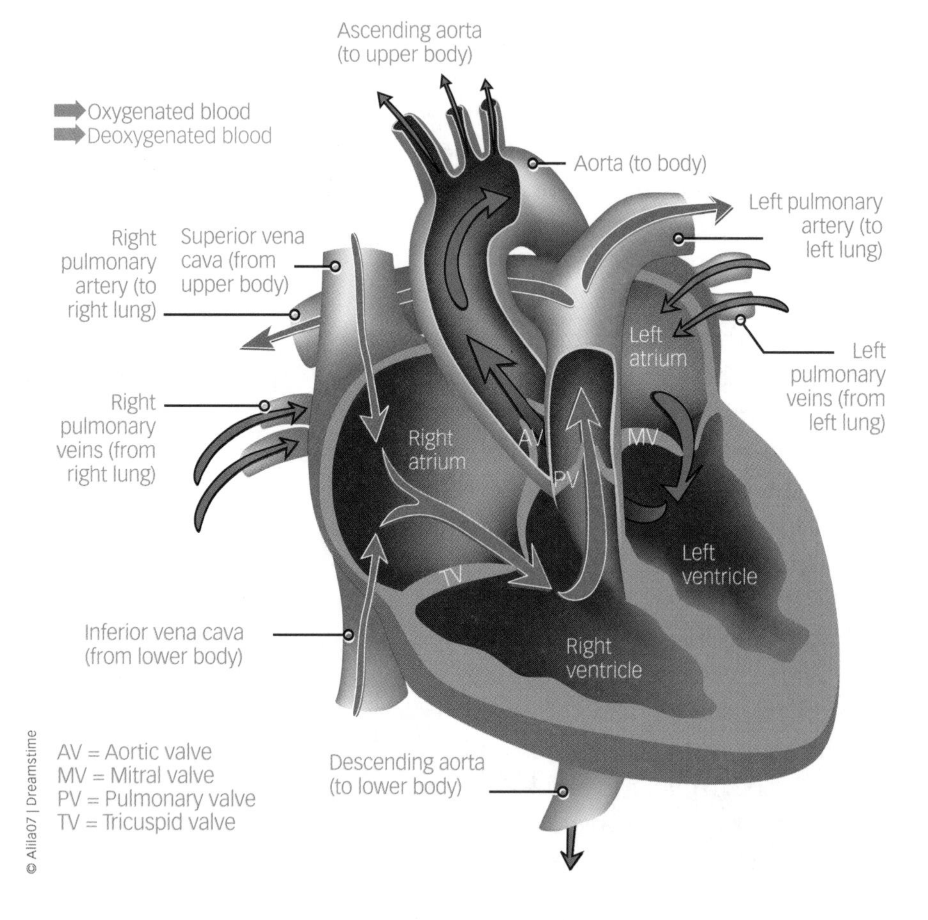

Your heart has two atria and two ventricles functioning as two parallel circulatory systems in your body. The right and left sides of your heart work in synchrony—while the ventricles are contracting, the atria are filling to prepare for the next cycle.

Pulmonary circulation system: The pulmonary circulation system involves the right side of the heart. This side pumps blood into the lungs to pick up oxygen and release carbon dioxide, a waste product produced by cells.

Peripheral circulation system: The peripheral circulation system uses the left side of the heart to pump oxygen-rich blood to the rest of the body.

shortness of breath. Although women are far less likely than men with systolic heart failure to die in the hospital, they are more likely to be discharged to a skilled nursing facility rather than to their home.

Causes of Heart Failure

Multiple medical problems can weaken the heart's ability to pump. By far the most common causes are heart attack, cardiomyopathy, hypertension (high blood pressure), and diabetes.

Heart Attack

A heart attack occurs when one or more arteries that nourish the heart muscle become blocked or narrowed by fatty deposits (plaque) or a blood clot. When the flow of blood slows or stops, the area of heart muscle fed by that artery does not receive nourishment from oxygen-enriched blood.

Atherosclerotic plaques can interfere with blood flow in two ways. In one form, they grow slowly, becoming hard and calcified over time and gradually reducing the diameter of the artery. Patients with hard plaques experience chest pain (angina pectoris) when they exercise, exert themselves, or consume a big meal.

Angina is a cramp in the heart muscle, which is a sign the muscle is not receiving enough blood. If it disappears with rest, it is called stable angina. Stable angina may be treated with medications to dilate and relax the arteries. But as the disease progresses, stable angina may become unpredictable and more frequent, and it may begin to occur at rest. This is called unstable angina, and it can be the precursor to a heart attack.

Unstable angina often is treated in the catheterization lab with balloon angioplasty and stenting, or by coronary artery bypass surgery. Even with treatment, however, a heart attack may occur. If it does, it may lead to a weakened heart muscle and heart failure.

Soft plaques that have a fatty core covered by a fibrous cap are even more dangerous than hard plaques. For

Circulation: Blood's Journey Through the Body

Oxygen-depleted blood returns from the body and enters the right side of the heart via the pulmonary veins. The right ventricle pumps blood out of the heart through the pulmonary valve into the pulmonary artery and the lungs. The tricuspid valve prevents the blood from leaking backward into the right atrium. The pulmonary artery divides into ever-smaller arteries until the blood vessels become microscopic in size. These are called capillaries, and in the lungs they surround tiny air sacs called alveoli.

Where the alveoli and capillaries meet, red cells in the blood give off carbon dioxide and pick up oxygen. Capillaries leaving the alveoli join into four pulmonary veins, which deliver oxygen-rich blood to the left atrium. After crossing the mitral valve into the left ventricle, the blood is pumped through the aortic valve into the aorta, the largest artery in the body.

The mitral valve prevents blood from being forced back to the lungs. The aorta divides into many arteries to distribute oxygen-rich blood throughout the body. It takes about 20 seconds for a red blood cell to make the journey from the heart through the body and back again.

The Lasting Legacy of a Heart Attack

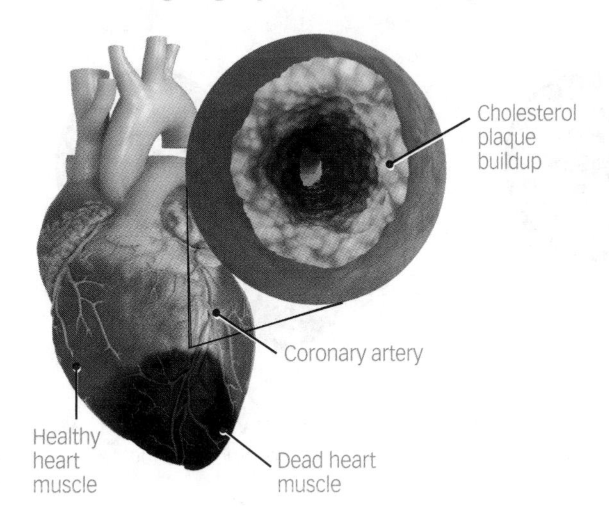

When oxygen-rich blood does not reach the heart muscle (myocardium) due to a cholesterol plaque buildup or a blood clot, tissue begins to die. This is a heart attack, and it can cause permanent damage to the muscle. Damaged tissue is not as pliable as healthy tissue—it cannot pump as efficiently, and sometimes it cannot pump at all.

reasons that are not entirely clear, the cap may rupture, releasing a variety of substances into the bloodstream that cause the blood to clot. If the clot blocks the flow of blood, a sudden heart attack occurs. Blood flow must be restored quickly to prevent part of the heart muscle from dying, causing scarring and permanent damage. Damaged areas of heart muscle are unable to contract—therefore, the heart cannot pump as strongly as it did before.

Cardiomyopathies

Up to half of all heart failure cases are caused by cardiomyopathies, which are diseases that primarily affect the heart muscle. Cardiomyopathies often occur without a known reason, but they also can be caused by various medical conditions, including infections (usually viral), metabolic disorders, endocrine disorders, and adverse reactions to medications. Cardiomyopathy may have an autoimmune or genetic component and also can be associated with alcohol or drug abuse, pregnancy, and prior radiation or chemotherapy.

Certain forms of heart failure appear to have a genetic basis. An analysis of participants in the long-running Framingham Heart Study showed a 70 percent increased risk of heart failure in people who had a parent with heart failure. In 10 years of follow-up, 2.7 percent of study participants with a family history of heart failure developed heart failure themselves, compared with 1.6 percent in those without a family history of heart failure. This means that people who have heart failure due to cardiomyopathy may want to encourage their children to be screened for the condition. The chance they have not inherited an increased risk of heart failure is very good. However, if early signs of heart failure are found, medications and lifestyle changes may be needed to delay its development (see

Known and Suspected Risk Factors for Heart Failure

The American Heart Association published a Scientific Statement on the prevention of heart failure that lists the following as established or hypothesized risk factors:

Major Clinical Risk Factors

- Age
- Male sex
- Hypertension (high blood pressure)
- Left ventricular hypertrophy (thickening of the left ventricle wall)
- Ischemic heart disease
- Myocardial infarction (heart attack)
- Diabetes mellitus
- Heart valve disease
- Obesity

Minor Clinical Risk Factors

- Smoking
- Anemia
- Dyslipidemia (a disruption in blood cholesterol or fats)
- Albuminuria (high levels of the protein albumin in the urine)
- Increased heart rate
- Diet
- Sleep-disordered breathing
- High blood levels of the amino acid homocysteine
- Chronic kidney disease
- Psychological stress
- Immune activation, IGF-1, TNF-alpha, IL-6, C-reactive protein (CRP)
- Natriuretic peptides
- Sedentary lifestyle
- Low socioeconomic status

Toxic Risk Factors

- Alcohol abuse
- Cocaine
- Chemotherapy agents: anthracyclines, cyclophosphamide, 5-FU, trastuzumab
- Nonsteroidal anti-inflammatory drugs (NSAIDs), such as aspirin and ibuprofen (Advil, Motrin)
- Thiazolidinediones, such as rosiglitazone (Avandia) and pioglitazone (Actos)

Genetic Risk Predictors

- Single-nucleotide polymorphism (a change to a single base in the DNA)

Morphological Risk Predictors

- Increased left ventricular internal dimension or mass
- Asymptomatic left ventricular dysfunction
- Left ventricular diastolic dysfunction

Atherosclerosis

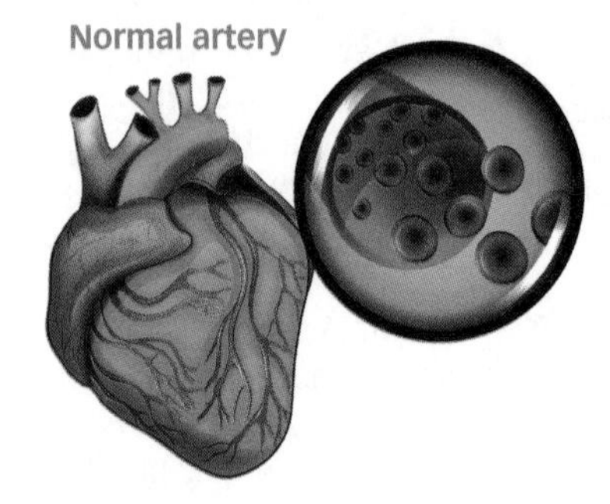

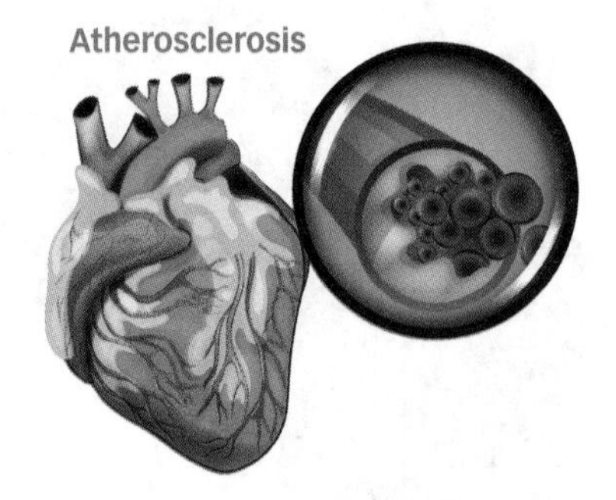

© Viktoria Kabanova | Dreamstime

In atherosclerosis, plaque deposits build up inside the artery walls. This narrows the arteries, meaning the heart has to work harder to force blood through a smaller channel.

"First Drugs for ATTR Cardiomyopathy Approved in 2019").

There are three major forms of cardiomyopathy, all of which may have a genetic component:

- **Dilated cardiomyopathy.** In this form, all chambers of the heart enlarge (dilate), and the ability of the left ventricle to contract is weakened. More blood than normal remains in the enlarged ventricle after a heartbeat, meaning that less blood is pumped out with each contraction.
- **Hypertrophic cardiomyopathy.** In this form, the muscle mass and thickness of the left ventricle walls increase, which makes the interior of this chamber smaller.

  In hypertrophic obstructive cardiomyopathy (HOCM), the wall between the two ventricles (septum) becomes enlarged and obstructs blood flowing out of the left ventricle. In non-obstructive hypertrophic cardiomyopathy, the thickened muscle does not obstruct blood flow and may contract vigorously, but it becomes stiff and is unable to relax normally. This causes improper filling between heartbeats: Less blood enters the ventricle, so less blood is pumped out. Improper filling causes blood to back up in the veins of the lungs, producing high blood pressure in the lungs (secondary pulmonary hypertension).

  Because of the strong genetic component of hypertrophic cardiomyopathy, anyone diagnosed with the disease should encourage their children and siblings to have an echocardiogram and, possibly, a genetic test, or at minimum, receive genetic counseling. Recent research indicates their risk of having heart failure or hypertrophic cardiomyopathy is 70 percent greater than normal.

  A medication for HOCM is now being tested in small human clinical trials. Early results have been encouraging, and larger studies are planned (see "Hope for First HOCM Drug").
- **Restrictive cardiomyopathy.** In this type of cardiomyopathy, the heart is stiff and cannot fill properly, even though its pumping strength may be normal. An insufficient amount of blood enters the heart, so too little is pumped out. This uncommon form of cardiomyopathy may be caused by abnormal scarring (fibrosis), abnormal infiltration of the heart muscle with iron (hemochromatosis) or protein (amyloid), or an unknown reason.

NEW FINDING

First Drugs for ATTR Cardiomyopathy Approved in 2019

In 2019, the U.S. Food and Drug Administration (FDA) approved the first two drugs for treating transthyretin amyloid cardiomyopathy (ATTR-CM), tafamidis meglumine (Vyndaqel) and tafamidis (Vyndamax). In ATTR-CM, which may be inherited or acquired, amyloid protein accumulates in the heart muscle, causing heart failure. The drugs work by slowing the formation of amyloid.

In studies leading to FDA approval, tafamidis significantly reduced hospitalizations and deaths without increased risk of adverse events. The 30-month mortality rate in people treated with tafamidis was 29.5 percent, compared with 42.9 percent in those treated with placebo.

FDA News Release, May 3, 2019

Hypertension

When the heart pumps, it pushes blood just like a weightlifter lifts a barbell. If there is little resistance, it's like a light barbell that requires very little effort. In hypertension, there is more resistance to the flow of blood through the arteries, so the heart has to work harder to push blood through the body. This is like adding weight to the barbell—and adding more weight makes the barbell harder to lift.

About 75 percent of people with heart failure have a history of hypertension, and the lifetime risk of developing heart failure with a blood pressure higher than 160/90 millimeters of mercury (mmHg) is double that of blood pressure lower than 140/90 mmHg. Although up to 90 percent of people age 80 and older have some degree of hypertension, it is not normal, and it greatly increases

NEW FINDING

Hope for First HOCM Drug

The first-in-humans clinical trial of a drug called mavacamten brings hope that an effective treatment for hypertrophic obstructive cardiomyopathy (HOCM) is in the near future. Patients with HOCM have increasing shortness of breath, fatigue, and chest pain as the walls of their heart thicken and begin to obstruct blood flow from the left ventricle to the aorta. In this open-label clinical trial of 21 symptomatic HOCM patients, mavacamten improved blood flow through the heart during exercise and at rest, lessening shortness of breath. The drug was well tolerated, with most adverse events considered mild. Clinical trials in larger numbers of patients will now follow.

Annals of Internal Medicine, June 4, 2019

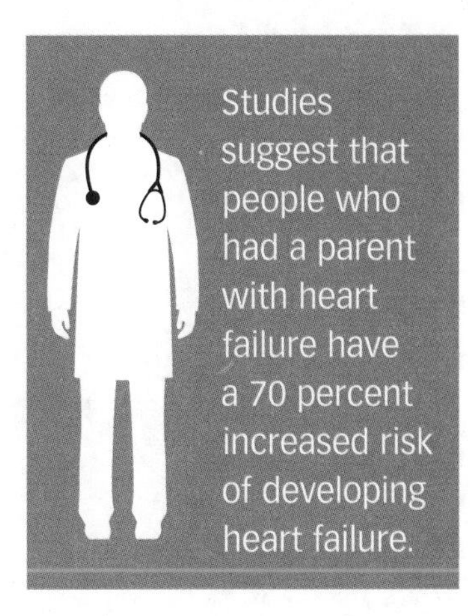

Normal Heart vs. Cardiomyopathies

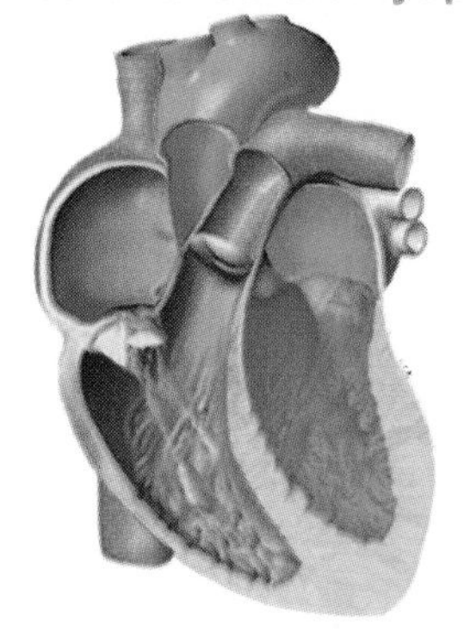

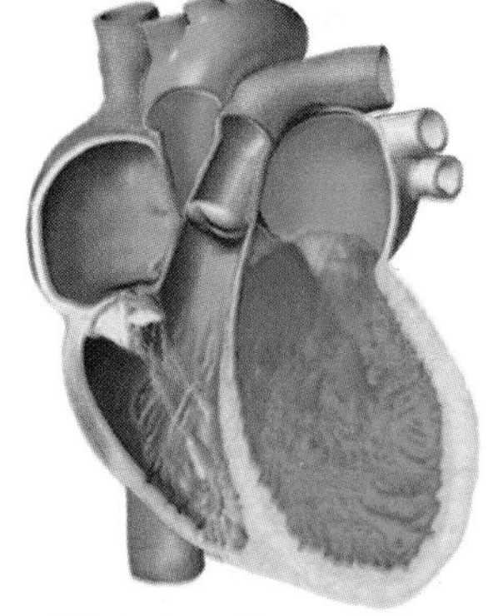

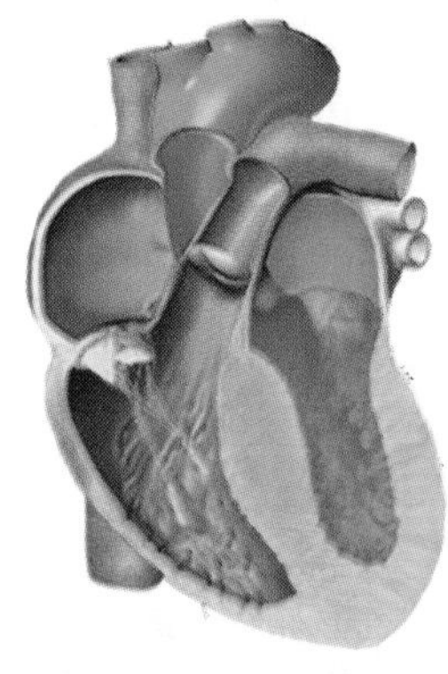

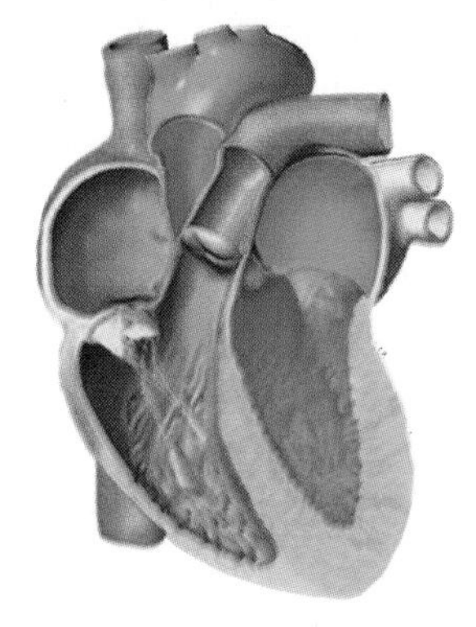

Cardiomyopathies are diseases that affect the heart muscle. They are believed to have a strong genetic component.

the risk of heart attack or stroke. Using medications to bring blood pressure below 120/80 mmHg can reduce the risk of heart failure, even in the very elderly.

Diabetes

Women with type 2 diabetes (the subtype that is common in older and obese adults) have a 2.4-fold increased risk of developing heart failure. Men with type 2 diabetes have a five-fold increased risk. The presence of other risk factors, such as coronary artery disease or hypertension, further increases the risk. People with diabetes or prediabetes who are hospitalized with heart failure have an increased risk of dying in the hospital and require intensive glucose control to lower the risk.

Type 1 diabetes (an autoimmune disease that typically develops during childhood) quadruples the risk of heart failure. When type 1 diabetes is poorly controlled, the risk is 10 times that of people without diabetes. Patients with kidney damage from diabetes as determined by their levels of albumin (a protein made by the liver) have an 18-fold higher risk of heart failure, even at a much younger age. For unknown reasons, women with type 1 diabetes have a higher risk of heart failure than men with type 1 diabetes. Although type 1 diabetes cannot be eliminated, patients with this disease can lower their risk of heart failure by maintaining very tight control over their blood sugar levels.

Other Causes and Risk Factors

Other causes of heart failure and risk factors that increase the chance of developing heart failure include valve disease, congenital heart defects, endocarditis (heart valve infection), myocarditis (inflammation of the heart muscle), persistent untreated tachycardias (rapid heart rhythms), obesity, anemia, malnutrition, and pregnancy. Certain medications and a variety of infectious agents, including common viruses and human immunodeficiency virus (HIV), also increase heart failure risk. So can diseases of the lungs, kidney, and liver. Too much thyroid hormone (hyperthyroidism) has been found to increase the risk of death from heart failure, even when levels were on the high side of normal or so slightly elevated that symptoms had not appeared.

More recently, researchers at Cleveland Clinic and elsewhere have identified a strong connection between bacteria in the intestinal tract and heart failure severity. All people with heart failure may have massive amounts of bacteria in their intestinal tracts, particularly when their heart failure is advanced. The types of bacteria that have been identified include *Campylobacter*, *Shigella*, *Salmonella*, *Yersinia enterocolitica*, and *Candida*. These patients also have increased levels of inflammation and intestinal permeability. High levels of intestinal bacteria indicate that a rise in intra-abdominal blood pressure and congestion in the circulation is causing edema (swelling) in the gut. This allows bacteria to leak out of the digestive system. According to Cleveland Clinic researchers, this finding confirms that a breakdown in the gut barrier is a result of heart failure, not a cause of it.

Some chemotherapy drugs given for cancer may be toxic to heart muscle cells and increase the risk of heart failure. These include doxorubicin (Adriamycin) and other anthracyclines, bevicizumab (Avastin), mitomycin (Mutamycin), mitoxantrone (Novantrone), sorafenib (Nexavar), sunitinib (Sutent), and trastuzumab (Herceptin), a monoclonal antibody approved for the treatment of metastatic breast cancer. The angiotensin-receptor blocker candesartan (Atacand), a common heart medication, may help preserve the heart's function in patients who have just begun taking anthracyclines. In 2019, researchers showed that people with heart failure caused by chemotherapy may benefit from cardiac resynchronization therapy, as well (see "Pacing Technique Overcomes Chemo-Induced Heart Failure").

Treatment with radiation to the chest for lymphoma, and breast, lung, or esophageal cancer also can result in heart failure, particularly when radiation is given in conjunction with one of the above drugs or given to people who have other risk factors for developing heart failure. Patients who take these chemotherapy agents should be considered at increased risk for heart failure and monitored regularly for signs of cardiac dysfunction.

Is Prevention Possible?

For the most part, heart failure is preventable. That's because it's often the

High Blood Pressure

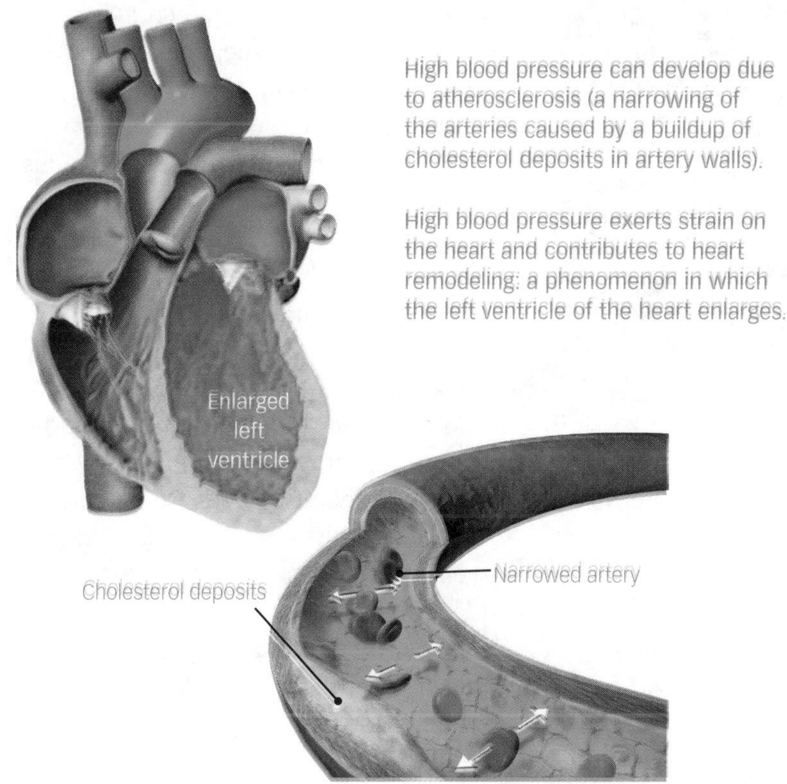

High blood pressure can develop due to atherosclerosis (a narrowing of the arteries caused by a buildup of cholesterol deposits in artery walls).

High blood pressure exerts strain on the heart and contributes to heart remodeling: a phenomenon in which the left ventricle of the heart enlarges.

Blood pressure is the force exerted on the walls of arteries by the blood as it circulates.

With each heartbeat, blood pressure experiences a maximum level (systolic, which is the upper number in a blood pressure reading) and a minimum level (diastolic, which is the lower number in a blood pressure reading).

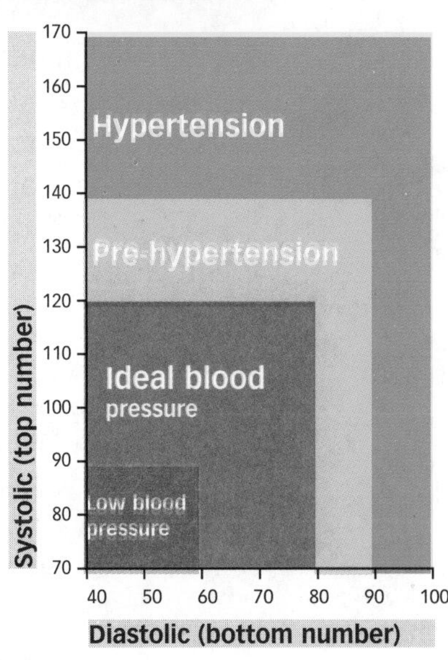

NEW FINDING

Pacing Technique Overcomes Chemo-Induced Heart Failure

It is particularly tragic when people survive cancer only to find that the medications that made this possible resulted in heart failure. The good news is that cardiac resynchronization therapy may help these individuals. Researchers implanted a biventricular pacemaker in 30 people with chemotherapy-induced heart failure. These pacemakers pace both sides of the heart to help it beat more efficiently. In six months, 29 study participants saw a significant improvement in ejection fraction, in essence reversing heart failure.

Annual meeting of the Heart Rhythm Society, May 2019

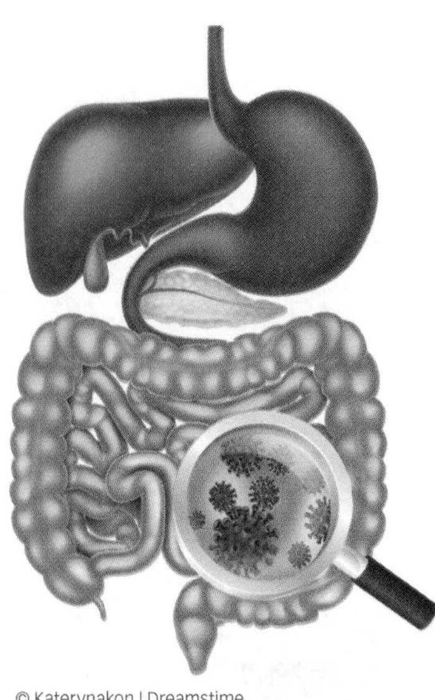

© Katerynakon | Dreamstime

Cleveland Clinic researchers have identified a strong connection between gut bacteria and heart failure severity.

result of another disease that can be prevented by managing underlying risk factors such as high blood pressure, coronary artery disease, obesity, and diabetes. This means taking measures to lower blood pressure, lose weight, control blood sugar, and avoid alcohol abuse and illicit drugs. It is particularly important in men and African Americans, who are more likely to develop heart failure than women and Caucasians.

Despite the myriad risk factors for heart failure—including those that can be modified and those that cannot—there is positive news in the American Heart Association's *Heart Disease and Stroke Statistics—2019 Update:* The one-year mortality rate from heart failure dropped slightly from 1998 to 2008, although it remains high, at 29.6 percent. The likelihood of dying varied widely among races and locations in the United States.

Lowering dangerous levels of triglycerides (fats that circulate in the blood) and low-density lipoprotein (LDL, also known as "bad" cholesterol) plays a major role in preventing coronary artery disease. However, low LDL and total cholesterol may be a marker of poor outcomes in heart failure patients. Studies of patients with cardiac cachexia (body-wide loss of muscle mass due to heart failure) and end-stage heart failure have shown that the likelihood of dying rises as total cholesterol levels fall. This challenges the theory that everyone with high cholesterol should take statins to lower it.

Despite this so-called "cholesterol paradox," heart failure patients who take statins may reduce their risk of heart attack and death by 20 to 25 percent. In another paradox, heart failure patients who are heavier and have slightly higher blood pressure actually do better than their thinner peers whose blood pressure is normal.

Early identification of patients with heart muscle dysfunction, which occurs before heart failure develops, allows for appropriate medical treatment that may prevent the progression of heart failure.

Stopping Further Deterioration

Once heart failure has started, heart function may never return to normal. For most people, the goal becomes to prevent their heart function from deteriorating further. This means taking medications, even when symptoms are absent or improve. The use of angiotensin-converting enzyme inhibitors and beta-blockers (see Chapter 7) or appropriate interventions—for example, replacing aortic valves narrowed by calcium deposits, or performing coronary bypass surgery (see Chapter 8)—can improve heart muscle function in select patients.

Advanced remote-monitoring techniques using internal and external devices appear to help prevent further deterioration by enabling physicians to intervene early to prevent hospitalization. One remote monitoring device reduced hospital admissions for heart failure by 43 percent and readmissions by 78 percent.

For the best care and latest techniques to maintain the heart's pumping power, getting treatment at a medical center with special expertise in heart failure is highly recommended. Recent studies clearly show that advanced multidisciplinary care can reduce hospitalizations and improve quality of life.

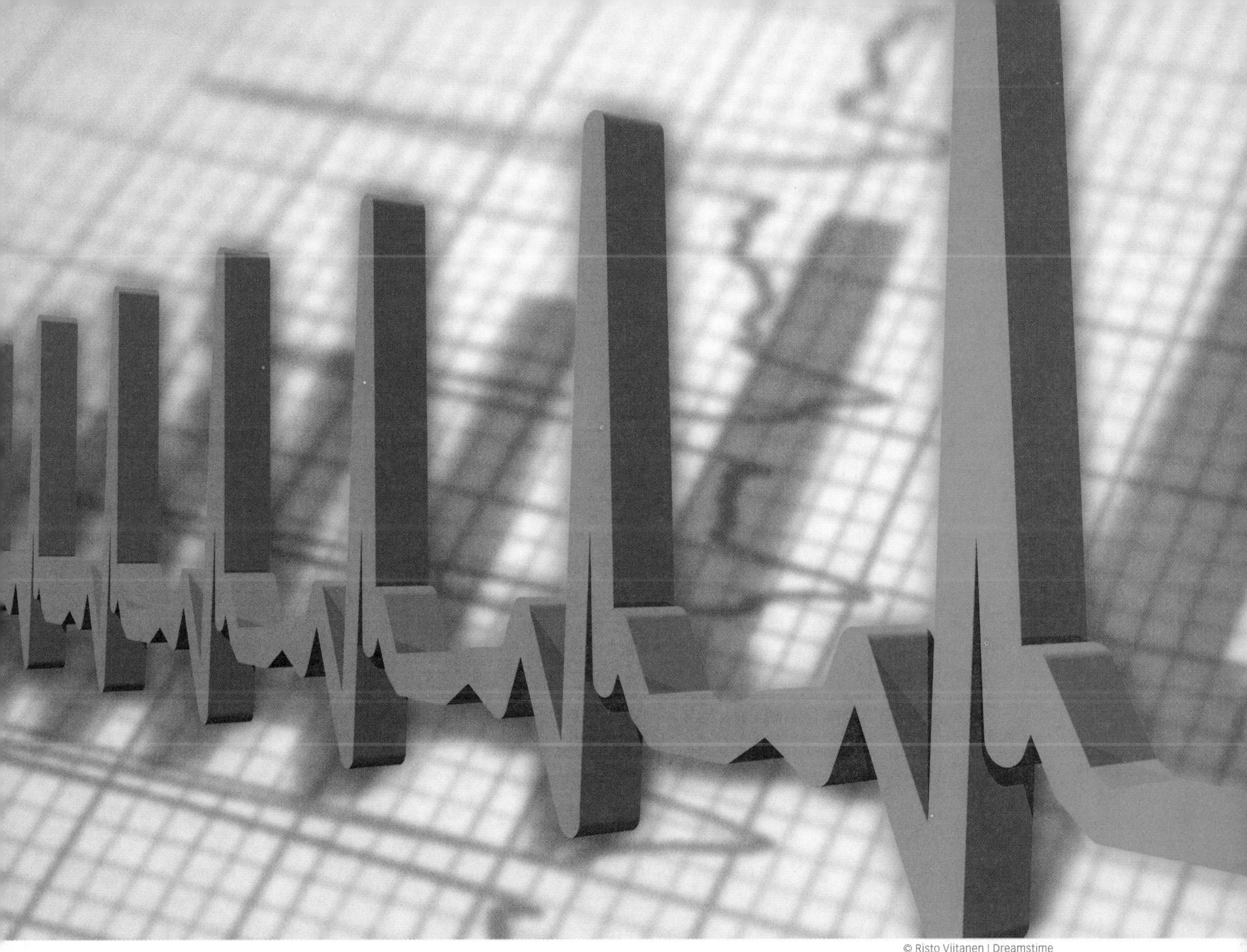

© Risto Viitanen | Dreamstime

An overworked heart is more likely to fail.

3 What Goes Wrong in Heart Failure

A normal heart is able to meet the body's demand for well-oxygenated blood. When that demand goes up, such as during exercise, the heart beats faster and stronger to increase the amount of blood being pumped through the body every minute. This is known as cardiac output. However, a heart that is failing has trouble meeting this demand and tries to compensate through a variety of complex metabolic, hormonal, and biochemical changes. At first, compensatory mechanisms prevent symptoms from manifesting. Over time, however, the heart's power and efficiency diminish to the point that it cannot supply the body's demand for blood and oxygen. This is when the early symptoms of heart failure begin to appear.

The Overworked Heart

In most forms of heart failure, the ventricles increase in size to compensate for weakened heart function. Heart muscle cells called cardiomyocytes lengthen and thicken, resulting in a stronger contraction that allows the heart to pump more blood with each beat. As the heart dilates, its chambers can fill with more blood, allowing the weakened heart to eject a normal volume with each beat.

However, the larger amount of blood entering the ventricles puts additional stress on the heart's walls, increasing

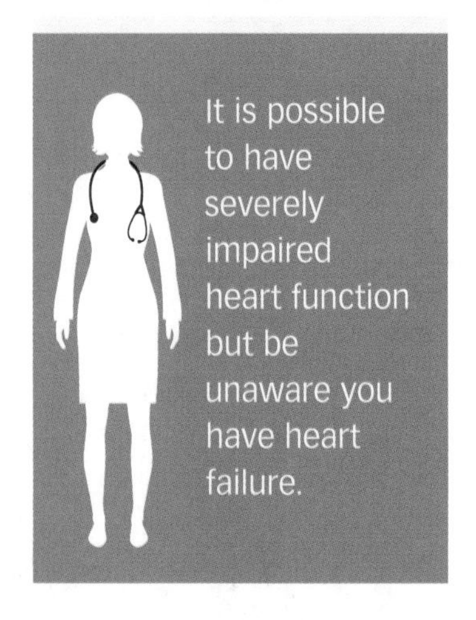

their demand for oxygen. The increase in pressure as the ventricles fill (filling pressure) causes blood to back up into the lungs. This in turn leads to too much fluid (congestion) in the lungs and the body.

The extra workload causes the heart muscle to thicken (hypertrophy), which occurs naturally with any muscle that is exercised. But unlike a bicep, a thickened heart muscle is not desirable. This is because as the heart walls become thicker, the heart demands more oxygen, and it becomes harder for the individual cardiomyocytes to relax.

These conditions cause the body to release various hormones, peptides, and inflammatory factors, all of which are described below.

Norepinephrine

The sympathetic nervous system, which automatically regulates heart rate and strength of contraction, reacts to the heart's struggle to pump by releasing norepinephrine. This neurohormone, which is related to adrenaline, accelerates the heart, increasing its demand for oxygen. The sympathetic nervous system also stimulates the blood vessels to constrict and direct blood toward vital organs. Veins constrict to increase the amount of blood the body sends back to the heart.

The role of heart rate in heart failure deaths is attracting attention. In 2014, Canadian researchers found that the risk of death rose along with heart rate. Among 10,000 people with heart failure, those with heart rates over 90 beats per minute had the highest risk of subsequent hospitalization for heart failure and risk of death at one year.

Renin-Angiotensin-Aldosterone

The renin-angiotensin-aldosterone system (RAAS), named for these three hormones, controls blood pressure and the amount of fluid in the body. When the heart is failing, the RAAS tries to compensate. The kidneys secrete a hormone called renin into the bloodstream. Renin converts a protein called angiotensinogen, which is produced continually by the liver and always present in the blood, to angiotensin I. When the blood carries angiotensin I to the lungs, it reacts with an enzyme called angiotensin-converting enzyme, forming yet another hormone called angiotensin II.

In the adrenal gland, angiotensin II triggers the release of still another hormone, called aldosterone. Aldosterone signals the kidneys to retain sodium and water from the bloodstream. This increases blood volume, which increases blood pressure. Aldosterone also causes the kidneys to excrete potassium.

Angiotensin II also interacts with its receptors on muscle cells of arterioles (small arteries), causing them to contract, thereby constricting the arterioles and hindering the flow of blood. Its effect is like pinching a water hose—it makes it harder for the same amount of water to flow through. In the case of blood vessels, the effect raises blood pressure, which increases the amount of work that the heart has to do.

This coping mechanism—which would be helpful in the short term if the body were actually dehydrated—leads to symptoms and signs that characterize heart failure:

- Swelling (edema)
- Shortness of breath (dyspnea)
- Congestion due to the body retaining salt and water.

As the number of angiotensin II receptors increases in heart failure, the body becomes more sensitive to the hormone's blood-pressure-raising effects.

Vasopressin

Vasopressin is a hormone produced in the hypothalamus gland to regulate water excretion by the kidneys when blood volume is low. People with heart failure typically have high levels of vasopressin. However, the body mistakenly senses that fluid levels are too low and produces vasopressin to increase the amount of water reabsorbed by the kidneys. Vasopressin also constricts blood vessels.

Endothelin

Endothelin is a peptide secreted by the cells lining the arteries (endothelium). The amount of endothelin present in the blood is directly related to the severity of heart failure. Endothelin is a powerful vasoconstrictor that may prevent the heart muscle from pumping effectively, and also promote abnormal heart rhythms (arrhythmias).

Cytokines

Proinflammatory cytokines (interleukin-1, interleukin-2, interleukin-6, and tumor necrosis factor-alpha) are peptides produced by cells in response to injury. They are found in increasing numbers in patients with atherosclerosis, and appear to play a key role in increasing the risk of cardiac events.

In heart failure, cytokines trigger a host of activities that cause myocardial (heart muscle) cell death, skeletal muscle dysfunction and wasting (cachexia), and weight loss.

A Phenomenon Called Remodeling

Over time, these neurohormonal changes lead to a phenomenon called remodeling, in which the left ventricle (the heart's main pumping chamber) becomes enlarged, and the individual heart muscle cells change size and shape. Having the walls of the heart stretch may be beneficial at first, but like an overstretched rubber band, they eventually become too stretched to contract very well.

Likewise, the increase in heart rate initially helps the heart pump out more blood. But since it raises the demand for oxygen in the heart muscle, over time it may lead to myocardial ischemia, which is an inability to deliver enough oxygen-rich blood to the heart muscle. Reduced blood flow to the inner layer of the heart muscle further impairs cardiac function. The increased heart rate has the potential to directly damage heart muscle.

Unless an attempt to restore balance is made, the vicious cycle continues. The heart works harder as it tries to compensate, and over time these efforts cause increasing harm. Eventually, heart failure may progress to the point where the heart can no longer compensate for the stresses placed on it. Breathlessness and fatigue become so severe that hospitalization is necessary. At this point, heart failure is said to be decompensated. To use the weightlifter analogy, the barbell has become so heavy that the weightlifter can no longer lift it.

The Remodeled Heart

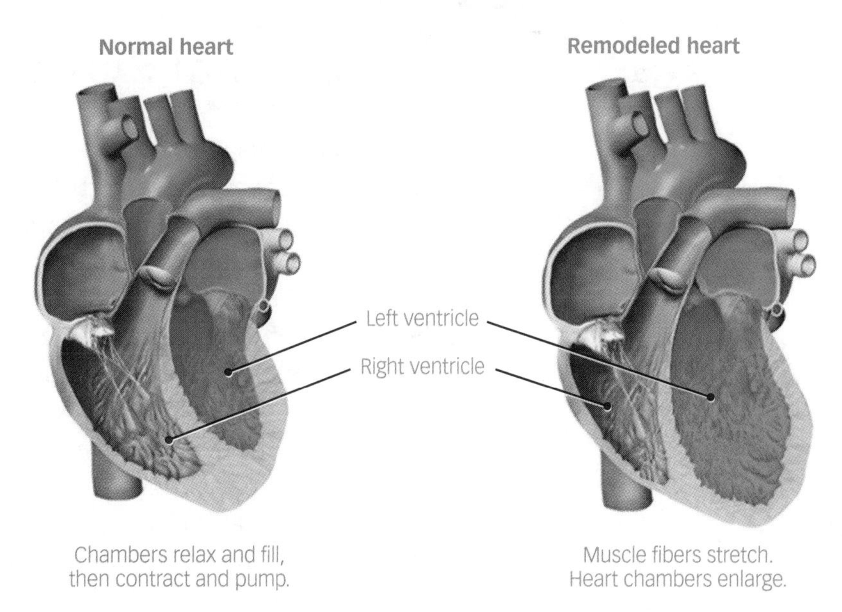

Many conditions can cause the heart to "remodel" itself in an attempt to compensate for injury or weakness. Remodeling increases the size of the heart's main pumping chamber and, subsequently, increases its workload. It also may increase backflow through the mitral valve (regurgitation), adding to the stress already placed on the abnormal heart muscle.

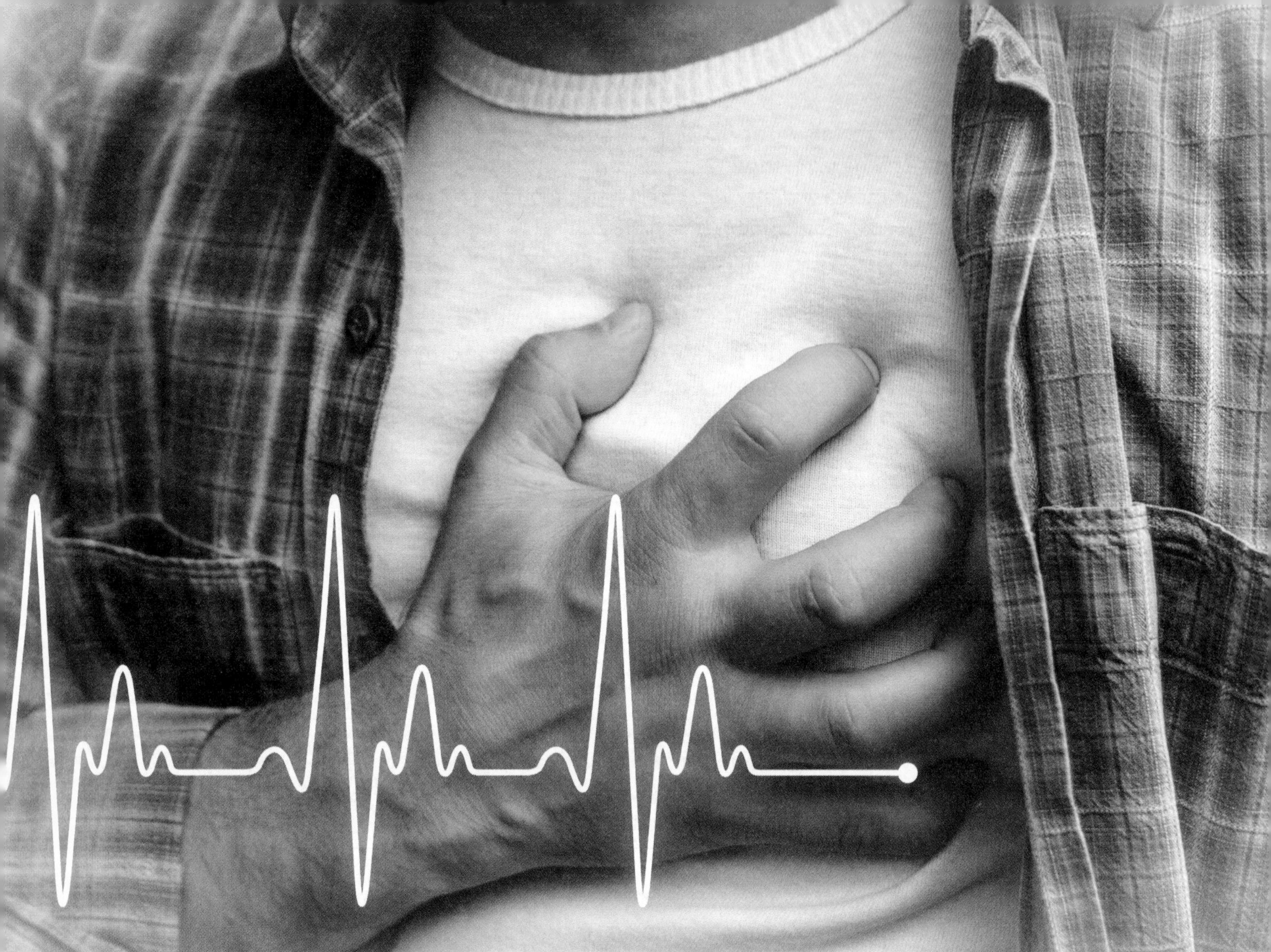

© Hriana | Dreamstime

A pounding heart can be a common symptom of heart failure.

4 The Usual Symptoms of Heart Failure

As the heart gets weaker, symptoms generally appear (although it is possible to have significantly impaired heart function and not know it). Symptoms may be mild or severe, depending on the severity of the heart failure and whether it affects the left or right side of the heart.

The left side of the heart receives oxygen-rich blood from the lungs, so when the left side of the heart fails, blood backs up into the lungs. This makes breathing difficult and can cause fluid to leak into the lungs, producing congestion (pulmonary edema). As more fluid is retained, the right ventricle may begin to fail.

In right-sided heart failure, blood coming into the right side of the heart from the body (the venous return) backs up. This causes excess fluid to pool in the legs and ankles, abdomen, and gastrointestinal tract. However, the location of the swelling can vary greatly.

Common Heart Failure Symptoms

In addition to affecting the heart, heart failure affects other organs in the body. The most common symptoms include:

- **Fatigue.** Because the heart muscle does not work effectively, the muscles of the body do not receive enough oxygenated blood. This causes fatigue and weakness, especially with exertion. Researchers have found that people with heart failure may feel fatigued for the same reason athletes who participate in endurance sports experience fatigue: After extreme exercise, such as running a marathon, calcium leaks into muscle cells, weakening the muscles. Until they recover, the athlete feels exhausted.

- **Difficulty breathing when lying down (orthopnea).** When you lie flat, blood from your lower extremities flows back to your heart. A weakened left ventricle cannot handle the increased volume, and blood backs up in the lungs, producing congestion and coughing. Patients with orthopnea must use pillows, a wedge, or a recliner chair to elevate their heads or upper torso to sleep.
- **Shortness of breath (dyspnea).** When fluid accumulates in the lungs, breathing becomes more difficult. Congestion causes rales, which are noises in the lungs that sound like crackles and can be heard with a stethoscope.
- **Shortness of breath when bending over (bendopnea).** Shortness of breath within 30 seconds of bending over is a sign of decompensation requiring more aggressive treatment, particularly in heart failure patients who are of normal weight or underweight.
- **Swelling (edema).** Excess fluid seeps through the blood vessel walls into the body tissues, primarily causing swelling in the legs and ankles, but also in the abdomen (ascites).
- **Difficulty sleeping.** Fluid buildup in the lungs may cause people with heart failure to awaken feeling short of breath (called paroxysmal nocturnal dyspnea), and they also may cough and wheeze.
- **Unusual weight gain.** If your heart failure worsens, you may experience a rapid weight gain of several pounds in a day or two from salt and water retention.
- **Poor circulation.** When blood is shunted to the vital organs to try to keep them functioning properly, this means that less blood flows to the hands, feet, and skin. Thus, the hands and feet look pale and feel cool, and the lips and fingernails may develop a blue tint (cyanosis).
- **Decreased urination.** In severe heart failure, the kidneys may not receive

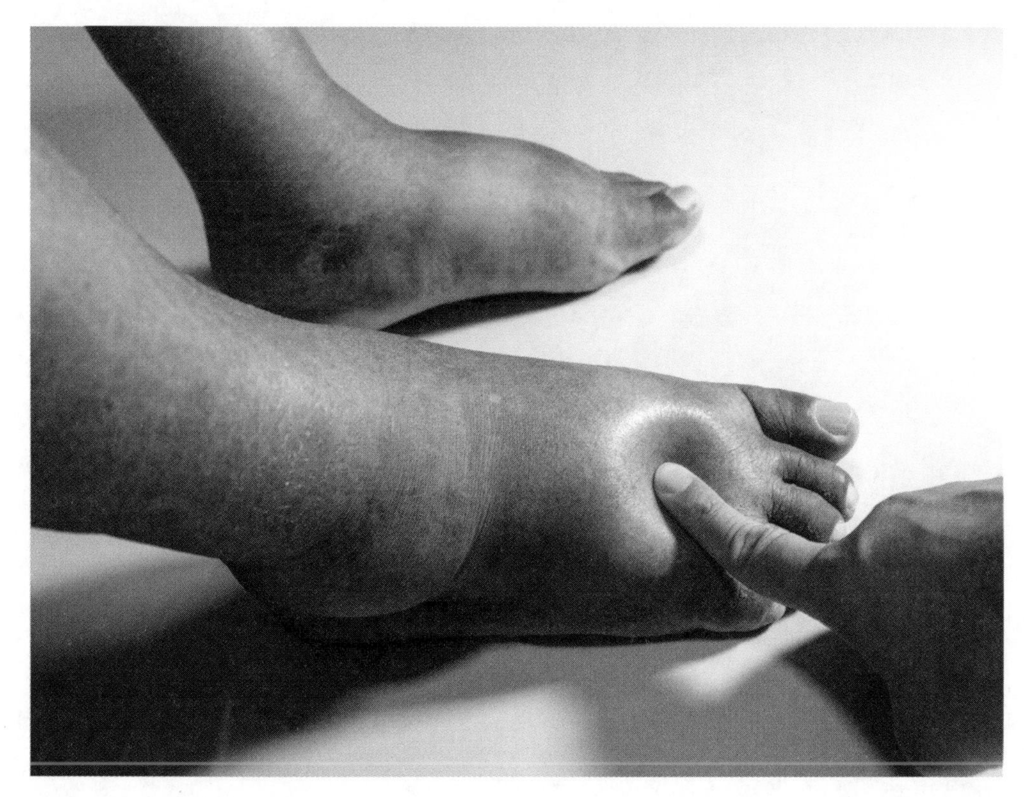

Heart failure typically causes swelling in the feet and ankles, but the abdomen also may be affected.

A Systemic Illness

Heart failure affects organs throughout the body, causing the following symptoms:

- Difficulty concentrating (brain)
- Shortness of breath (lungs)
- Generalized weakness (muscles)
- Bloating, poor appetite (abdominal organs)
- Increased or decreased urination (urinary tract)
- Muscle weakness (legs)
- Swelling (legs and abdomen)

enough blood to make urine. As a result, urine production may decrease.

- **Lightheadedness and dizziness.** As your heart failure worsens, you may experience abnormal heart rhythms or low blood pressure (hypotension). Either of these may cause you to feel lightheaded and dizzy.
- **Abdominal bloating.** Fluid retention may result in a tender or swollen abdomen, nausea, bloating, and a poor appetite.
- **Irregular heart rhythm (arrhythmia) or pounding heart.** Heart failure may produce a change in the pattern or efficiency of the electrical signals in your heart. This may cause a variety of arrhythmias that may be particularly noticeable when you are laying on your left side.
- **Impaired mental processes.** Low cardiac output may cause poor memory, drowsiness, and confusion. These symptoms may indicate that your heart failure is getting worse.

If your heart failure symptoms become less frequent or less severe, it may indicate that you are doing all the right things and your heart is performing as well as it can. If so, it's important to let your doctor know. It also is wise to tell your doctor if the frequency or severity of any symptom increases. It might mean that your heart failure is getting worse, and your doctor may want to adjust your medications.

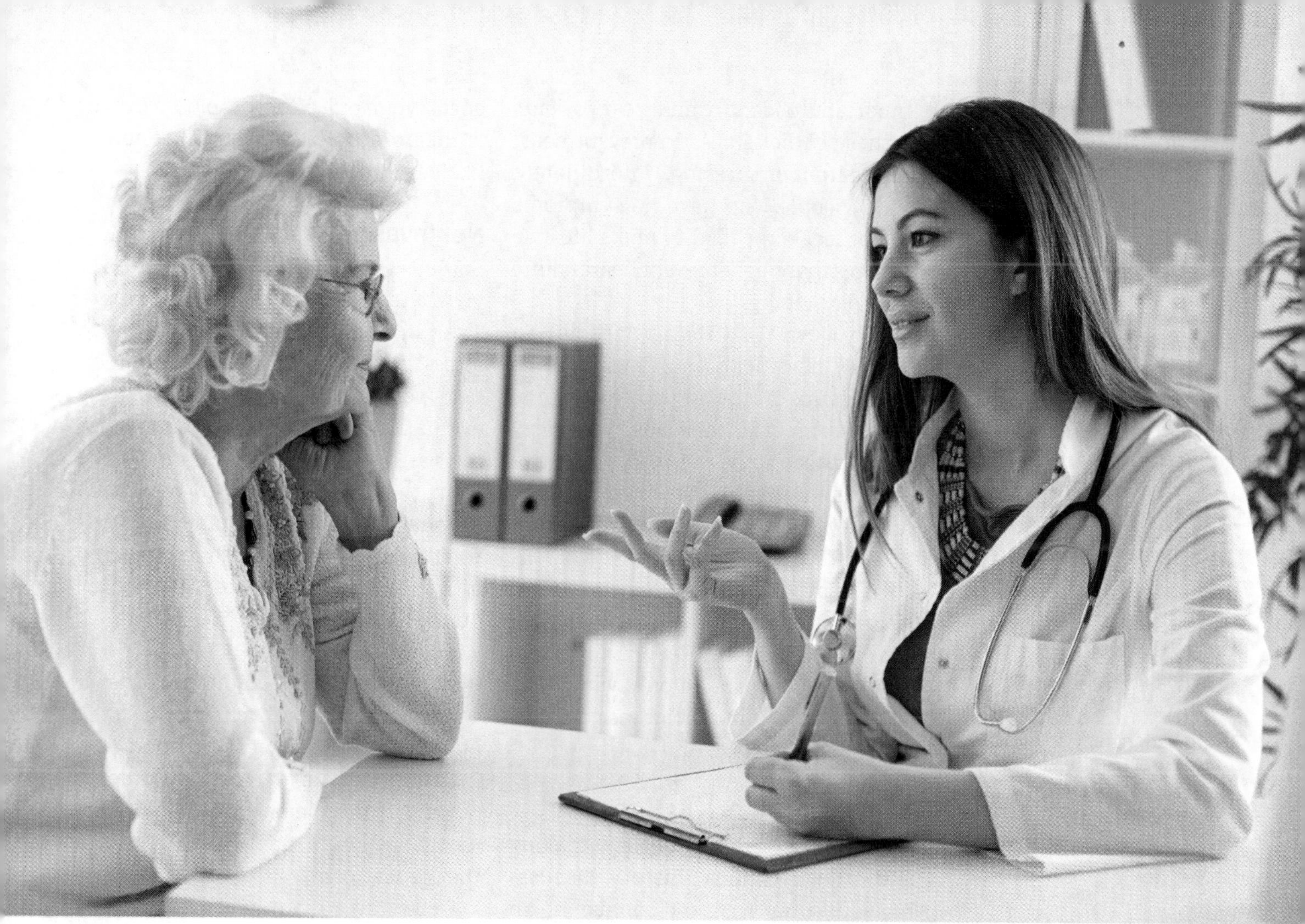

© Didesign021 | Dreamstime

Your cardiologist will regularly evaluate how well your treatment plan is working.

5 Diagnosing Heart Failure

An accurate diagnosis is essential for devising and implementing the most effective heart failure treatment plan. Your cardiologist will want to identify the underlying cause of your heart failure, assess how severely your heart's function is impaired, and determine how serious your condition is.

If you have been diagnosed with heart failure, you will need to see your cardiologist regularly to determine if your condition is improving, remaining stable, or progressing. Each visit is an opportunity to review your treatment plan and make any necessary adjustments.

Classifying Heart Failure Severity

Two complementary systems are used to classify heart failure severity. The American College of Cardiology (ACC) and the American Heart Association (AHA) classify heart failure based on the evolution and progression of the disease. Once a person advances to the next stage, he or she is unlikely to move backward. The ACC/AHA system links each stage to recommended treatments.

The ACC/AHA system also broadens the scope of classification to include people who are at risk for developing heart failure, and those who have structural heart disease but no symptoms. This is an important distinction, because these individuals should be advised and treated accordingly.

When treatment is started before heart failure symptoms appear (ACC/AHA stages A and B), it reduces the risk of complications or death. Therefore, it is

ACC/AHA Stages of Heart Failure

- **Stage A.** At high risk for heart failure, but without structural heart disease or symptoms of heart failure.
- **Stage B.** Structural heart disease, but no signs or symptoms of heart failure.
- **Stage C.** Structural heart disease with prior or current symptoms of heart failure.
- **Stage D.** Refractory heart failure requiring specialized interventions, such as mechanical circulatory support, continuous inotropic infusions, cardiac transplantation, or hospice care.

NYHA Functional Classification of Heart Failure

- **Class I (No Impairment).** No limitation of physical activity. Ordinary physical activity does not cause symptoms of heart failure.
- **Class II (Mild-to-Moderate).** Slight limitation of physical activity. Comfortable at rest, but ordinary physical activity results in symptoms of heart failure.
- **Class III (Moderate).** Marked limitation of physical activity. Comfortable at rest, but less-than-ordinary physical activity causes symptoms of heart failure.
- **Class IV (Severe).** Unable to perform any physical activity without symptoms of heart failure, or symptoms are present at rest.

important to identify and treat patients in these earlier stages to prevent heart failure from progressing. Unfortunately, many people who have no symptoms do not feel compelled to make lifestyle changes that might prevent heart failure from developing.

The New York Heart Association (NYHA) classification divides patients into groups according to the degree of impairment in their ability to carry out physical activity. It is a subjective assessment made by the physician, and represents a patient's condition at the time of evaluation. A patient's NYHA class may change between visits as treatments take effect or the disease progresses. The NYHA classification system is comparable only with ACC/AHA stages B, C, and D; there is no NYHA equivalent for stage A.

Tests for Heart Failure

Your cardiologist will begin by taking a thorough medical history, discussing your symptoms, and conducting an extensive physical examination. Using a stethoscope, he or she will listen for abnormal sounds (such as murmurs) that reveal problems with your heart's function. A stethoscope also will allow the doctor to hear crackling sounds (called rales) that indicate fluid in the lungs. The cardiologist will check your neck for distended neck veins, feel your abdomen for signs of fluid retention and liver enlargement, evaluate your skin color, take your blood pressure, and check your pulse for a rapid or irregular heart rate. Blood and urine tests will likely be ordered.

Biomarkers Commonly Used in Heart Failure

Multiple biomarkers can be used to help establish or rule out heart failure, determine its severity, track clinical status, and identify adverse reactions to treatment.

BIOMARKER	IDENTIFIES
Natriuretic peptide	Myocardial stretch, heart failure
Cardiac troponin	Myocyte injury, heart attack
C-reactive protein	Inflammation
Creatinine	Renal dysfunction
BUN	Renal dysfunction

Noninvasive Tests

Some tests will enable your doctor to view and measure your heart's shape, size, function, and capacity to respond to stress and exercise. The most common tests you are likely to have during the evaluation are discussed below. These tests are essentially noninvasive—apart from the probe swallowed for transesophageal echocardiogram, and contrast agents or radionuclides injected into a vein, nothing enters your body during the tests.

Blood Tests. Your doctor will order a complete blood count, chemistry panel, lipid profile, and thyroid-function test. In addition, your doctor may order a blood test for one or more biomarkers, most of which are proteins released into the bloodstream.

Detecting a biomarker in the blood can be helpful in making the diagnosis of heart failure and assessing its severity. Studies have shown that the combination of two or more biomarkers may be even better at predicting a person's risk of heart failure. In some cases, this allows a cardiologist to make better treatment decisions. Levels of these biomarkers are significantly higher in patients who have heart failure than in patients with normal hearts.

Chest X-Ray. A chest x-ray can reveal changes in the heart's size and shape, as well as the presence of congestion in the lungs, sometimes before any heart failure symptoms appear.

Electrocardiogram (ECG or EKG). An ECG provides information about the heart and its electrical function. Sticky electrodes placed on the arms, legs, and chest record the heart's electrical activity from different angles as it signals different areas of the heart to contract and relax. This painless test usually lasts less than a minute.

An ECG can:

- Detect evidence of a previous heart attack and show what part of the heart was affected.
- Determine whether an underlying heart rhythm abnormality (arrhythmia) is contributing to heart failure.
- Indicate whether a chamber of the heart is enlarged.
- Show thickening of the heart muscle due to hypertension, cardiomyopathy, or a valve disease, such as aortic stenosis.

Doctors use an ECG to measure the width and duration of QRS waves, which indicate the time it takes for electrical activity to spread throughout the ventricles. The QRS duration can be used to determine whether someone may qualify for a biventricular pacemaker.

The combination of an ECG and stress test can be used to screen for coronary artery disease, determine functional capacity, and check for abnormal heart

Chest X-Ray

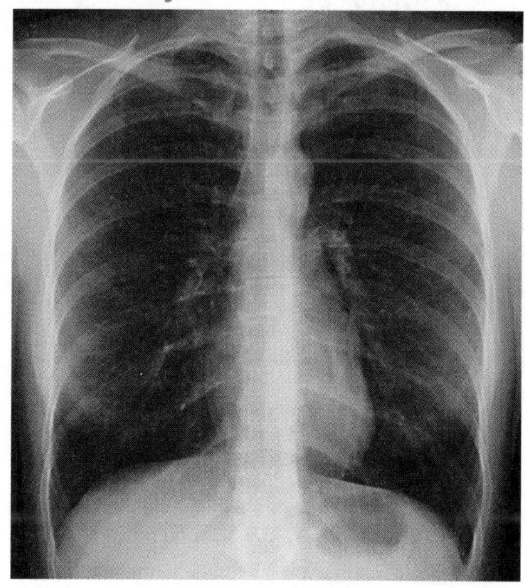

A chest x-ray shows the trachea (airway), heart (center), lungs, and diaphragm, as well as the collarbone, ribs, and spinal vertebrae.

The Electrocardiogram Recording

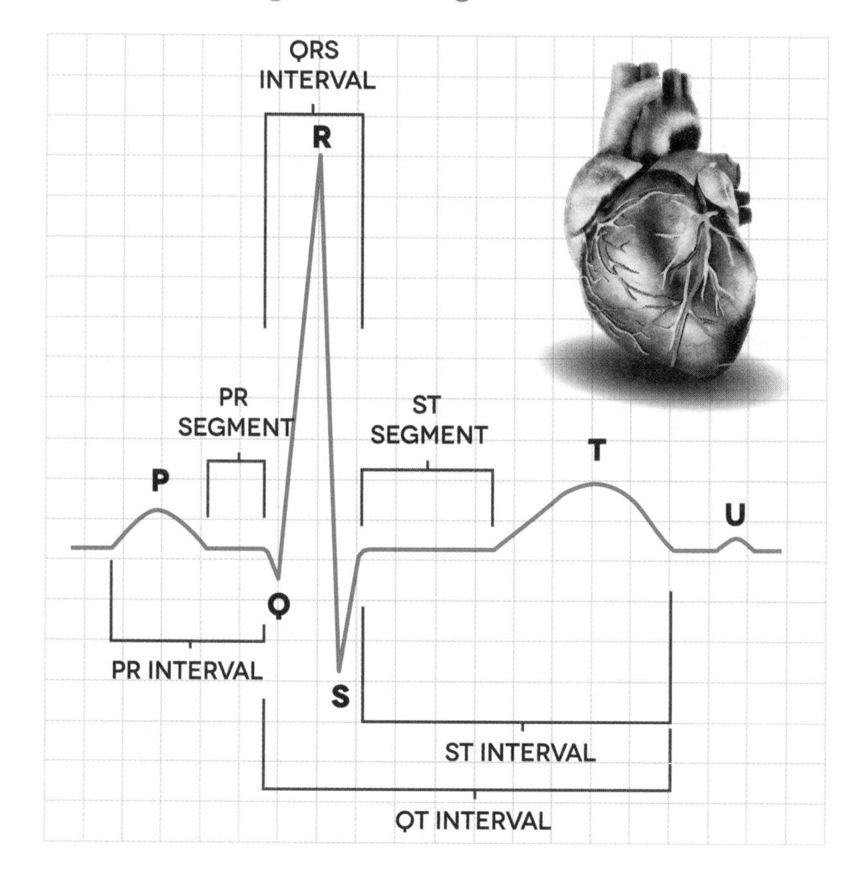

Heartbeat Waves

The normal heartbeat can be distinguished on an electrocardiogram (ECG) by a series of electrical oscillations called P, Q, R, S, and T waves.

The first recorded electrical oscillation is called the P wave; it is the impulse that stimulates atrial contraction. A series of three waves—the Q, R, and S waves—is the impulse that stimulates ventricular contraction. The T wave represents the relaxation of the ventricular muscle.

A normal heart rate is considered to be 60 to 100 beats per minute. The duration of the ECG cycle is about two-thirds of a second, and it becomes even shorter as the heart beats faster during exercise. A particularly narrow QRS interval reflects an abnormally fast heart rate.

Changes in the shape of the normal ECG tracing are an important diagnostic tool. For example, an elevated ST-segment is indicative of a heart attack, while peaked T waves along with a reduced P wave indicate hyperkalemia (elevated potassium levels that can cause potentially fatal abnormal heart rhythms).

Echocardiogram and Doppler Echocardiogram

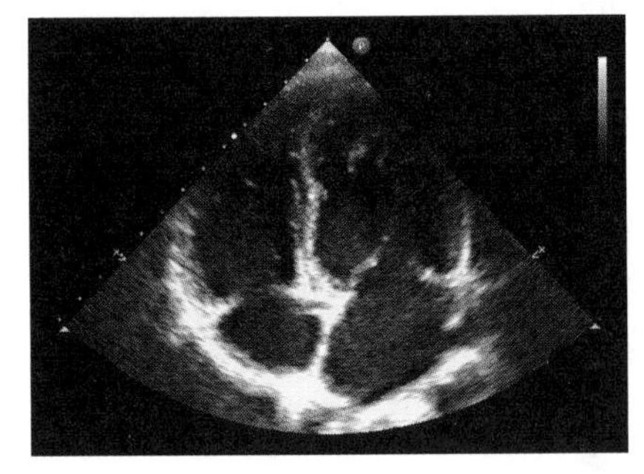

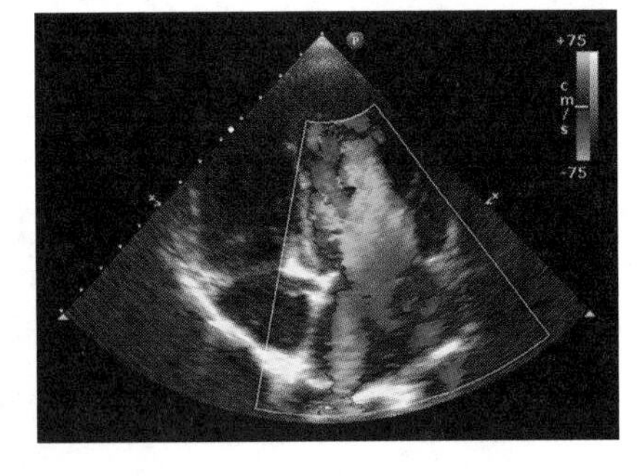

© Kalewa | Dreamstime

An echocardiogram (left) provides an image of the heart beating in real time, while a Doppler echocardiogram (right) also assesses blood flow through the heart.

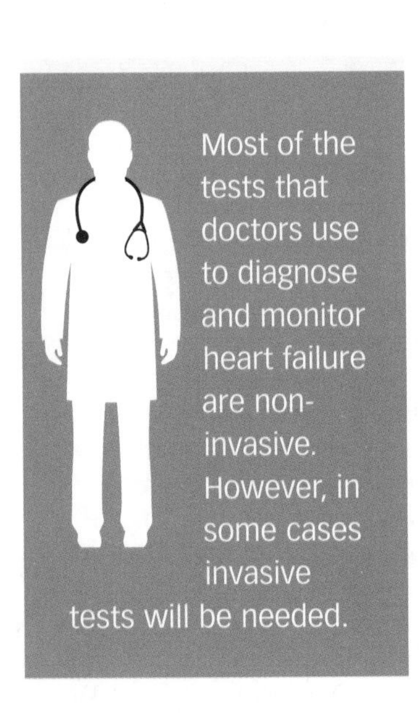

rhythms. ECGs are an important part of your health history. Your doctor will keep records of your past ECGs and compare them to see how your heart may have changed. If you have coronary artery disease or have had an abnormal ECG, you may want to carry a laminated copy of your latest ECG in your wallet or purse in case of an emergency. For extra safety, write the name and phone number of your cardiologist on the back.

Echocardiogram. An echocardiogram is an ultrasound that reveals the beating heart in real time. It can show the shape, size, position, and motion of cardiac structures, including the thickness of the ventricle walls. Echocardiograms also can show leaky (regurgitant) or narrowed (stenosed) heart valves, as well as abnormal openings between the chambers (septal defects).

Your cardiologist will use the results of your echocardiogram to calculate your ejection fraction, a key measure of how well your heart is functioning. Perhaps because of the importance of ejection fraction, and the fact that it is easily understood, you may be tempted to follow your ejection fraction closely and worry if it has not improved since the previous test. However, this tendency places too much importance on a number that can vary by as much as five percentage points either way on the same day. This variation occurs in part because of the many variables in cardiac testing.

It helps to think of the ejection fraction as an estimate, rather than a precise measurement. It is best to think of it in broad terms as mildly, moderately, or severely abnormal. When your ejection fraction increases or decreases, ask your doctor whether you are still in the same heart-function range as on your previous visit, or whether something has changed.

Like an ECG, an echocardiogram is painless and noninvasive, so there is no need for anesthesia or sedation. Sometimes, however, a contrast agent is used to improve image quality in patients who are obese or have lung disease.

To conduct the test, several electrodes are applied to the chest. A gel is then applied to a handheld echo probe (transducer), which is pressed against the chest. The probe sends and receives ultrasound waves, which bounce off the heart. A computer translates these sound waves into pictures. The images, which are generally stored on a computer, can be paused at any time during the heartbeat so the physician can measure the heart and its structures.

There are several different types of echocardiogram:

- **Doppler echocardiogram.** This is a regular echocardiogram that also assesses blood flow by measuring changes in the frequency of sound waves. During this test, you may hear a "whooshing" sound. This is not your blood flowing, but rather a computer reconstruction of the sound waves. Doppler echo is particularly useful in assessing the heart's valves.
- **Transesophageal echocardiogram (TEE).** This type of echo provides a closer look at the heart. It involves swallowing a small transducer (similar to a microphone). Once in the esophagus, the transducer is positioned next to the heart. Better images of the heart can be obtained from inside the body than

from the outside, especially for certain parts, such as the left atrium. TEE is most often used to assess complicated valve problems or the presence of blood clots. Although the test is generally not painful, patients are usually sedated, and the throat is numbed with a local anesthetic.

- **Exercise or stress echocardiogram.** This type of echo is used to determine the presence of coronary artery disease. A baseline echo is performed. The patient then exercises on a treadmill or stationary bicycle while the heart's response is carefully monitored. The rate of exercise, controlled by the speed and incline of the treadmill, is gradually increased until the heart is working very hard. When the patient cannot exercise any longer, another echocardiogram is taken. The test will show whether significant coronary artery disease has caused ischemia (decreased flow of blood) with exercise. A stress echo test also can be done with a contrast agent to improve image quality.
- **Dobutamine stress echocardiogram.** This type of echo is used for people who are unable to exercise or undergo stress echocardiography. A baseline echo is performed at rest. Then the drug dobutamine (Dobutrex) is given intravenously to make the heart work harder, as if it were exercising. The test may be used to assess coronary artery disease and valve disease, and to distinguish between scar tissue and viable heart muscle.

Metabolic Stress Test. Also called a cardiopulmonary exercise test, this is done on a treadmill or bicycle. This test is used to measure your functional capacity and how well you utilize oxygen during exercise.

During the test, you will wear nose clips so that only mouth breathing is possible. A mouthpiece will measure how much oxygen you inhale and how much carbon dioxide you exhale. Your peak oxygen consumption will be calculated and compared with what is normal for someone of your age, size, and physique. This provides an objective measure of the degree of functional impairment.

Radionuclide Stress Test. When a stress test is combined with the use of a radioactive isotope (usually thallium and/or sestamibi) injected into a vein, it is called a nuclear stress test, myocardial perfusion scan, or SPECT scan.

SPECT stands for single-photon emission computed tomography—"single-photon" because the isotopes emit only a single type of radiation (gamma rays). A special camera captures the gamma rays and a computer uses them to construct an image—hence, the test is "computed." Tomography is a method of reconstructing images in sections or planes. This enables a physician to look at a specific section of the heart to see how much blood it is receiving.

When the isotope is injected, the blood carries it to the heart, where it accumulates in areas with adequate blood flow. If a coronary artery is blocked, the isotope can't get through.

Multiple-Gated Acquisition Scan. A multiple-gated acquisition (MUGA) scan captures the heart in motion. A small amount of thallium or technetium is injected into a vein, and as the isotope flows through the heart, the size and shape of the ventricles and their pumping ability can be seen. This test helps assess how well the heart contracts, and measures the ejection fraction of both

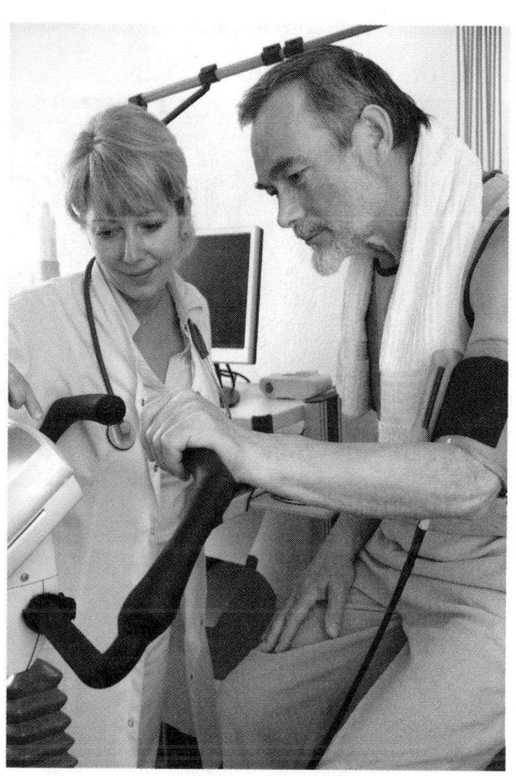

During a stress test, your heart rate will be monitored while you exercise.

Positron Emission Tomography

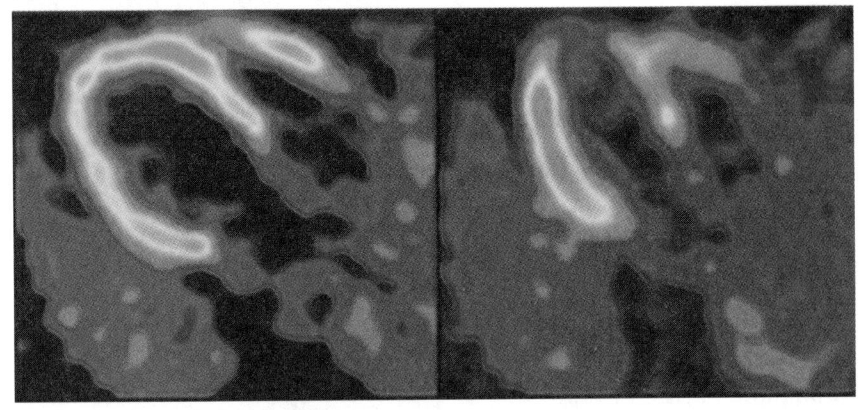

© openi.nlm.nih.gov

Positron emission tomography is used to identify areas of scar tissue in the heart muscle after a heart attack.

the left and right ventricles. The test may be done at rest or while exercising.

Positron Emission Tomography. Positron emission tomography (PET) is similar to SPECT, except that positron-emitting radionuclides are detected instead of gamma rays. PET is commonly used to differentiate between tissue that is metabolically active (alive) and tissue that shows no metabolic activity (dead). After a heart attack, PET can be used to identify dead tissue or scar tissue in the heart. When a heart attack has killed cardiomyocytes (muscle cells), they turn into scar tissue that cannot be restored.

Injured cardiomyocytes do not contract well, but they are alive and may revive if blood flow is restored. This condition is called "hibernating myocardium." PET can be used to identify regions of the heart that are likely to revive if blood flow is restored. In this respect, it is useful in determining whether a patient is a candidate for revascularization with stenting or coronary artery bypass grafting.

Magnetic Resonance Imaging

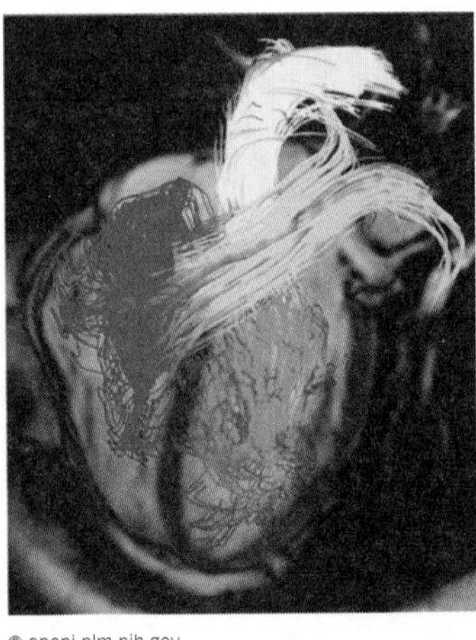

© openi.nlm.nih.gov

New developments in diagnosing and managing heart failure include four-dimensional (4D) magnetic resonance imaging, which allows for the comprehensive evaluation of complex blood flow patterns through the heart.

Magnetic Resonance Imaging. Magnetic resonance imaging (MRI) sometimes is used to obtain a detailed anatomical picture of the heart. MRI is particularly useful in assessing the health of the heart muscle, including the presence of a dangerous infiltrative protein, such as amyloid, scar tissue from past heart attacks, or hibernating myocardium.

An MRI is generally performed while the patient lies on a table that is eased into a long, tube-like scanner. (Some MRI units have an open design that accommodates heavy patients and those who are claustrophobic.) The test is painless—in fact, there is no sensation at all—but it can be noisy, as the machine makes banging sounds.

An MRI test uses powerful magnets and radio waves to produce images by recording energy emitted by cells when they react to the magnetic field. A computer analyzes these movements and creates a composite image of the tissues. Multiple pictures of the heart are taken from many angles. The computer uses them to construct detailed views of the heart, either still or in motion, in two, three, or four dimensions.

Because of the strong magnetic field exuded by the unit, many people with older pacemakers, defibrillators, or any implant containing iron cannot have an MRI. Newer cardiac devices are MRI-compatible.

Coronary Computed Tomography Angiography. Fast multi-detector computed tomography (CT) scanners (128- and 256-slice scanners with dual-source technology) enable doctors to obtain clear images of the heart and coronary arteries in seconds. CT provides an increasingly complete assessment of cardiac anatomy and function. The test requires an injection of a contrast agent and takes only seconds to complete.

Whereas traditional angiography performed during cardiac catheterization reveals the lumen, or empty space inside the artery, CT angiography clearly shows both the lumen and the artery wall. As such, it enables physicians to identify early plaques. CT technology may replace the need for the more invasive cardiac catheterization when the diagnosis of coronary artery disease is uncertain. For example, CT can be used for patients with chest pain and risk factors for heart disease who have had a negative stress test but who remain concerned about coronary artery disease. CT also can be helpful in patients with few risk factors for coronary artery disease who present to the emergency department with chest pain, and may be useful in evaluating patients with suspected dilated cardiomyopathy.

Physicians are still trying to determine which patients are the best candidates for CT angiography. Diagnostic accuracy is limited in patients with heavily calcified plaque or stents. Therefore, it cannot be used to assess in-stent restenosis (the re-narrowing of an artery after treatment with a stent). Although CT image resolution is fairly good in other types of patients, it is not good enough to replace cardiac catheterization before angioplasty or bypass surgery.

Pulmonary Function Tests. A pulmonary function test called spirometry can determine how well the lungs are working. Spirometry may be ordered to investigate whether shortness of breath is due to another cause that mimics heart failure. This simple test requires breathing into a tube attached to a machine that calculates the amount of air the lungs can hold and the rate at which it is inhaled and exhaled. The results are compared with those of healthy individuals of the same gender and similar height and age.

Invasive Tests

Invasive tests require a tube or sensor to be inserted into one of the blood vessels in the groin, arm, wrist, or neck. These tests, which are performed in a cardiac catheterization room (often referred to as a "cath lab"), are used to assess pressures in the heart and lungs, as well as cardiac output, coronary anatomy, and left ventricular function.

Cardiac Catheterization. In cardiac catheterization, a thin, flexible tube called a catheter is inserted into a blood vessel and advanced into the heart. The procedure is done under mild sedation. First, a local anesthetic is gently injected in the skin to numb the area in the groin, arm, or wrist, and a short tube with a valve on one end (sheath) is inserted in the artery

Computed Tomography

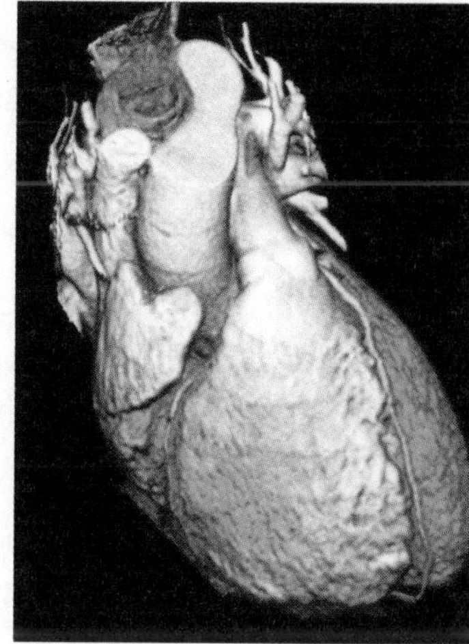

Computed tomography uses x-rays to create detailed images of the heart.

Cardiac Catheterization

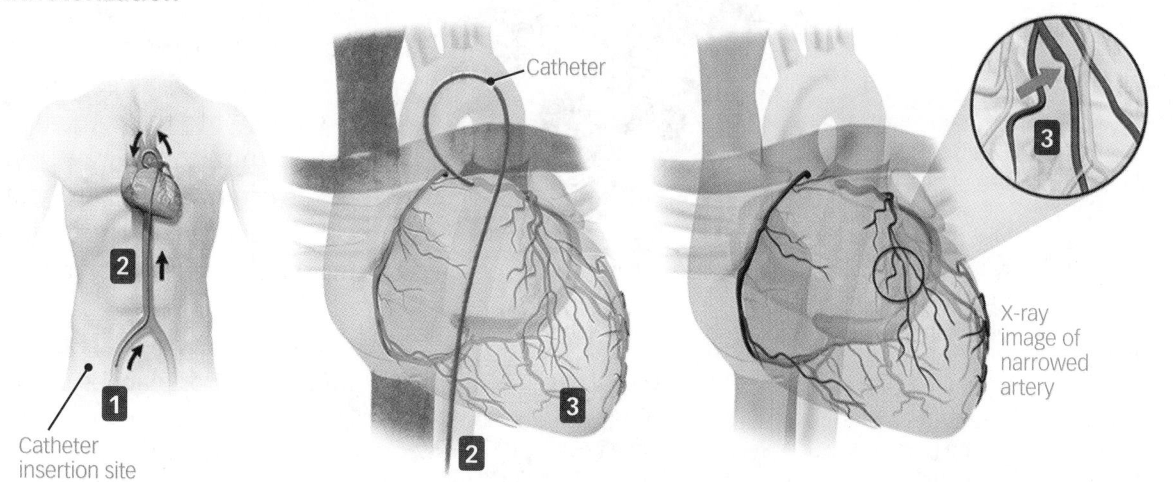

In cardiac catheterization, a flexible tube is inserted into a blood vessel (1) and guided to the heart (2) to determine the condition of the coronary arteries (3).

or vein. A catheter is introduced through the sheath and painlessly threaded to the heart.

The left side of the heart usually is catheterized shortly after heart failure is diagnosed, to determine the condition of the coronary arteries. The catheter is advanced into the aortic root, where the opening of the left coronary artery is located. At this point, a contrast agent (or "dye") is injected into the artery. An x-ray movie (angiogram) is taken to visualize the artery's appearance. The process is then repeated in the right coronary artery.

In a right-heart catheterization, the catheter is advanced into the right atrium, and then into the right ventricle and the pulmonary artery. Blood pressures in the pulmonary artery and right-heart chambers are recorded. A computer attached to the catheter calculates the amount of blood flow, which is equivalent to the amount of blood flowing through the body, as all blood passes through the pulmonary artery as it circulates. The results of this test are useful in helping a cardiologist adjust the medications used to treat heart failure. This test also is required for patients who are being considered for heart transplantation.

Electrophysiology Testing

In an electrophysiology (EP) study, an electrophysiologist inserts a recording catheter into a vein in the patient's groin and advances it to the right atrium (1) near the bundle of His (2), a band of fibers that conducts electrical signals (the bundle was named after its discoverer, Wilhelm His, a German cardiologist), and the right ventricle (3). Electrodes in the catheter transmit information about the heart's electrical activity. The doctor uses this information to evaluate the heart's electrical system and pinpoint the source of the arrhythmia. Programmed electrical stimulation is then used to deliver electrical signals through the catheter to increase the heart rate.

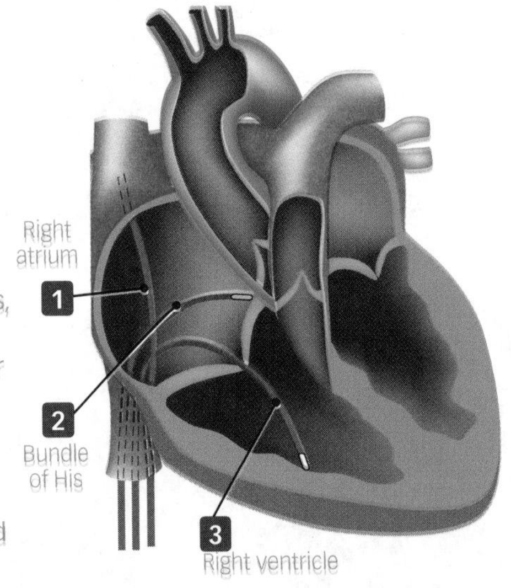

If an arrhythmia occurs, the doctor will intravenously administer anti-arrhythmic medication and evaluate the drug's ability to stop the arrhythmia. Based on the findings of the EP study, the doctor may decide to conduct an ablation procedure or implant a pacemaker or implantable cardioverter defibrillator. In ablation, high-frequency radio waves are sent through a special catheter to scar the abnormal cells causing the arrhythmia. The scarred area disrupts the passage of abnormal electrical impulses through the heart.

Ventriculography. During this procedure, a contrast agent is injected into the left ventricle, and images are taken and recorded digitally. The results of this test reveal the size and shape of the left ventricle, mitral regurgitation (leakage of blood back through the mitral valve), and how well the ventricle is pumping (ejection fraction).

Electrophysiology Testing. Electrophysiology testing (EP) is done to detect heart-rhythm problems, which can accompany heart failure. EP tests measure the heart's electrical impulses more thoroughly than other electrical conduction tests, and are sometimes performed to determine if a pacemaker or defibrillator is needed. EP tests may be done in a catheterization laboratory or a specially equipped electrophysiology laboratory.

Intravascular Ultrasound. Intravascular ultrasound (IVUS) is used when angiography does not provide enough information about the extent of coronary artery disease. In IVUS, a miniature transducer is snaked into the coronary arteries to bounce ultrasound waves off the walls of the artery. Signals are sent back to a computer that constructs pictures showing the artery, its walls, and the thickness of its lumen.

IVUS clearly reveals the shape, size, and density of plaques, as well as their composition. Learning whether a plaque is filled with soft, fatty cholesterol or hard calcium deposits can help your doctor determine the best type of treatment. If a blocked coronary artery is found, it may be treated with balloon angioplasty and a tiny metal support tube (called a stent) to keep the artery open. IVUS also may be used during or after an interventional procedure or medical therapy to track results, and also is used after heart transplantation to visualize the coronary arteries.

Myocardial Biopsy. In a myocardial biopsy, a special catheter with tiny jaws is guided to the right ventricle of the heart and a small piece of tissue is taken for examination. This test helps determine if the heart muscle has been infiltrated by white blood cells, fibrous tissue, protein, or iron. It may be used to investigate whether heart failure is caused by inflammation. This test is not often required for heart failure patients, but is used routinely to look for early signs of rejection in transplanted hearts.

Devising a Treatment Plan

Once you have been diagnosed with heart failure, your cardiologist will tailor a treatment plan to your condition. There are many components of the successful treatment of heart failure, and the best treatments for you will depend on what is causing your condition.

For people without symptoms, heart failure treatment focuses on preventing remodeling of the heart, holding off the development of symptoms, and minimizing risk factors for ventricular dysfunction and heart failure. In people who have symptoms, the goals are to improve quality and length of life.

Keep in mind that some of the components of heart failure treatment are under your control—and taking responsibility for improving your health can help you psychologically as well as physically. While medications and surgery may slow the progression of heart failure, it is up to you to provide a healthy environment for your overworked heart.

Intravascular Ultrasound (IVUS)

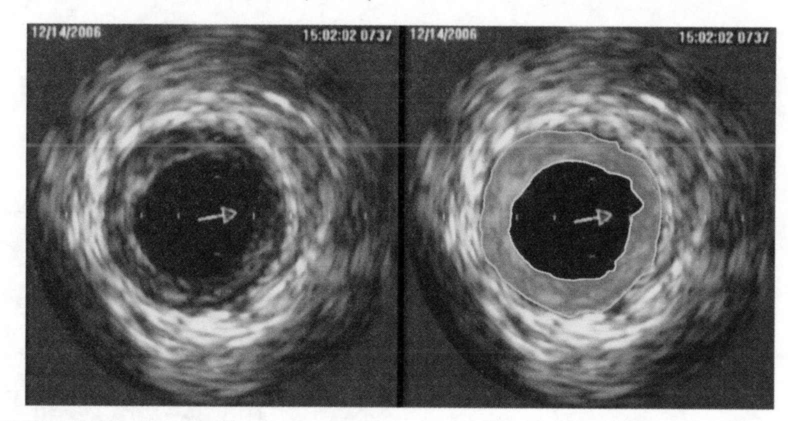

IVUS can reveal the shape, size, and density of arterial plaques, as well as clarify whether they are formed from soft, fatty cholesterol or hard calcium.

What Is a Stent?

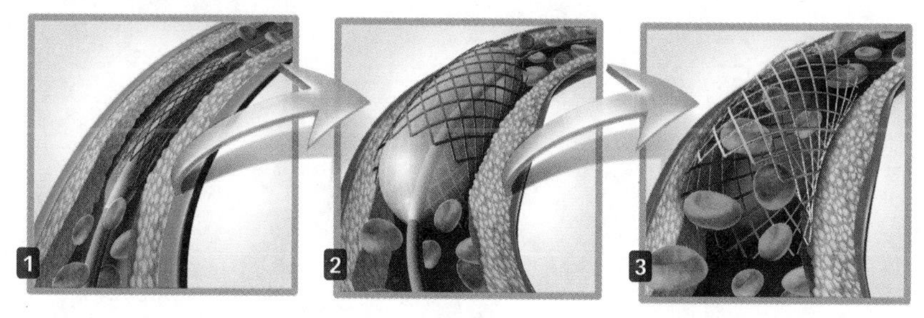

A stent is a tiny mesh tube that is inserted into a narrowed artery during a procedure called angioplasty. Once in position, the stent widens the artery and improves blood flow.

In stent deployment, a collapsed stent on a balloon catheter is threaded to the area of the plaque (1). The balloon is inflated, expanding the stent and pressing it against the plaque, causing a slight bulge in the artery (2). The balloon is then deflated and the catheter is removed, leaving the opened stent in place (3).

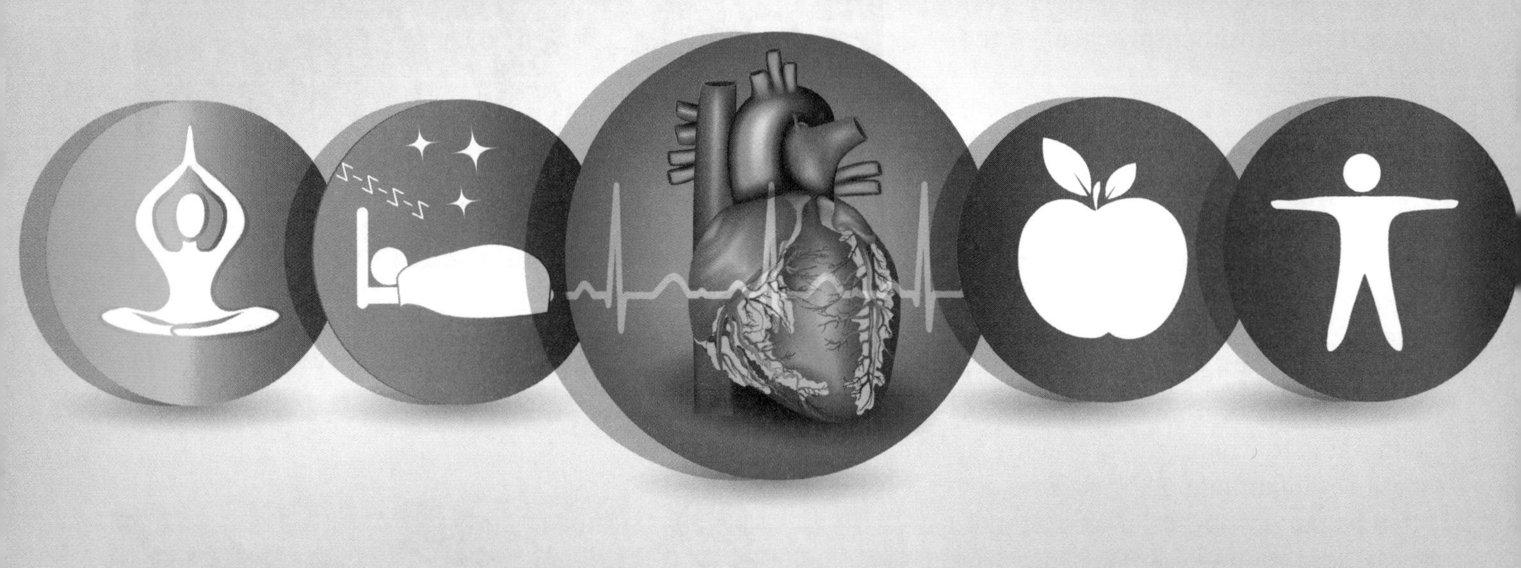

© Guniita | Dreamstime

Self-help strategies for managing heart failure include taking care of your mental health, getting sufficient sleep, eating a healthy diet, and staying physically active.

6 Heart-Healthy Lifestyle Changes

There are many steps you can take to slow the progression of heart failure and improve your quality of life. Start by breaking or avoiding unhealthy habits and engaging in healthy practices. Simple changes may enable you to lead a nearly normal life.

Nevertheless, living with heart failure can be a challenge. It takes teamwork and commitment to minimize symptoms and prevent the condition from progressing. You and your doctor must work together to keep your heart pumping as strongly as possible. Your doctor will provide you with instructions, and you must follow these instructions carefully to avoid shortness of breath, excessive fluid buildup, weight gain, and fatigue—and, ultimately, prevent your condition from worsening.

Since heart failure often is caused by a heart attack, reducing the chance of another heart attack will help lower the likelihood that your heart failure will worsen. This can be as easy as following what the American Heart Association calls "Life's Simple 7:" maintaining three blood markers within normal levels (blood pressure, blood sugar, and blood lipids) and practicing four healthy behaviors (quit smoking, eat better, get active and exercise regularly, and lose excess weight).

Achieving even five of the Simple 7 measures may reduce your risk of heart-related death by as much as 78

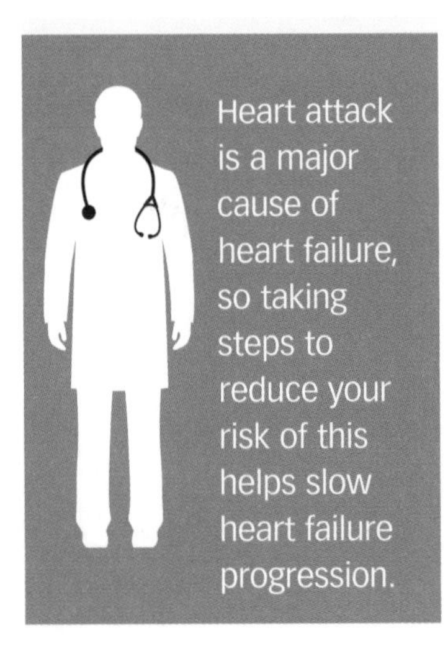

percent. How you can best follow them, along with other heart-healthy strategies, is covered in this chapter.

Quit Smoking

Smoking is the leading preventable cause of death in the United States, and smoking-associated deaths often are caused by heart attack.

Tobacco in any form (cigarettes, cigars, pipes, and chewing tobacco) wreaks havoc on the cardiovascular system, and smokers are two to three times more likely than nonsmokers to die from a heart attack. The good news is that when smokers quit, their risk of heart attack drops up to 50 percent after one year. After five years, their risk reaches that of a never-smoker.

When you finally decide to quit smoking, experts suggest you set a quit date within the next seven days and quit on that day. Success is more likely if you plan in advance how to deal with your cravings and urge to smoke. Most people find it extremely difficult to stop smoking on their own or to quit "cold turkey"—in fact, research suggests that the average person tries to quit the habit as many as seven times before succeeding. Using proven stop-smoking aids—nicotine-replacement therapy (patch, gum, spray, lozenges, or inhaler), cessation programs that incorporate hypnosis or acupuncture, or prescription medications, such as varenicline (Chantix) or buproprion (Zyban)—can reduce the number of unsuccessful attempts. A combination of methods—for example, the nicotine patch, a prescription medication, and counseling—increases the likelihood of success.

Experts also advise being physically active or using another form of stress management, such as yoga or meditation, and getting a buddy to help your transition into a nonsmoker. Try to avoid worrying about gaining weight after quitting: The few extra pounds are often temporary, and are far less of a health risk than smoking.

You are more likely to successfully quit smoking if you combine counseling with the use of smoking cessation aids.

Eat Better

Following a balanced, heart-healthy diet is essential. A diet high in omega-3 fatty acids (the kind found in fatty fish) has been shown to help prevent body wasting, a risk factor for death from heart failure. Studies also suggest that a diet high in whole grains may lower the risk of heart failure. Limiting sugary drinks, sweets, fats, fatty or processed meats, and highly processed foods also is recommended. Partially hydrogenated oils and tropical oils should be avoided. In addition, everyone with heart failure should limit the amount of salt and fluids they consume.

The Dietary Approaches to Stop Hypertension (DASH) diet and a Mediterranean-style diet are both good choices for patients with heart failure. When researchers looked at the effects of these diets on participants in the long-running Women's Health Initiative study, both diets were found to offer protection against death from heart failure.

Restrict Your Salt Intake

Limiting salt in your diet is one of the most effective ways you can manage heart failure, as well as your overall heart health. Salt contains sodium, which causes cells to retain water. Drinking excessive amounts of fluid increases blood volume, which can cause swelling (edema) and shortness of breath. Your kidneys may not eliminate water and salt as efficiently as a healthy individual's kidneys do. Your body also makes more renin, vasopressin, and aldosterone, which are hormones that increase salt and water retention. The result is a heart that works harder than it should.

A 2015 review of salt studies suggests that salt may harm other organs, as well. Various studies concluded that consuming large amounts of salt affects the lining of arteries and makes them stiff, harms the kidneys, blunts the effects of the "fight-or-flight" response, and may even impact the brain.

Sodium is found in many foods, most often in the form of sodium chloride (table salt). The average American consumes two to three teaspoons of sodium a day, much of it in prepared or processed foods. Your doctor will tell you how much sodium you can safely consume each day. Cleveland Clinic cardiologists agree with the Heart Failure Society of America's recommendation that consumption stay below one teaspoon a day.

Following a low-sodium diet requires more effort than merely avoiding adding salt. It's important to learn how much sodium is in the foods you buy and order in restaurants, and which foods are naturally low in sodium. It is equally important to learn which foods are very high in sodium and should be avoided. The American Heart Association calls the worst offenders "The Salty Six." They include cold cuts and cured meats, pizza, soup, breads and rolls, sandwiches, and burritos and tacos.

Understanding the following terms found on food labels will help:

- **Sodium-free:** Contains less than 5 milligrams (mg) of sodium per serving.
- **Very low sodium:** Contains 35 mg or less per serving.
- **Low sodium:** Contains 140 mg or less per serving.
- **Unsalted/no salt added:** Made without added salt but may still contain sodium that is naturally present in the food.
- **Healthy:** Contains 360 mg of sodium or less per serving.

Table salt isn't the only source of dietary sodium; other salts are used in cooking and food preparation. Baking soda and baking powder contain sodium bicarbonate. Some artificial sweeteners contain sodium saccharin. Many food preservatives and antioxidants are sodium-containing salts, such as sodium benzoate, sodium propionate, sodium ascorbate, and sodium erythorbate. Food thickeners and stabilizing agents used in ice cream, coffee creamers, and other foods include sodium caseinate and sodium carboxymethylcellulose. A teaspoon of soy sauce contains 700 mg of sodium.

"Lite" salt substitutes include sodium in reduced amounts, but those amounts are still too high for people with heart failure. It's important to talk to your

The DASH diet is designed to help lower blood pressure.

© Dmitry Rogatnev | Dreamstime

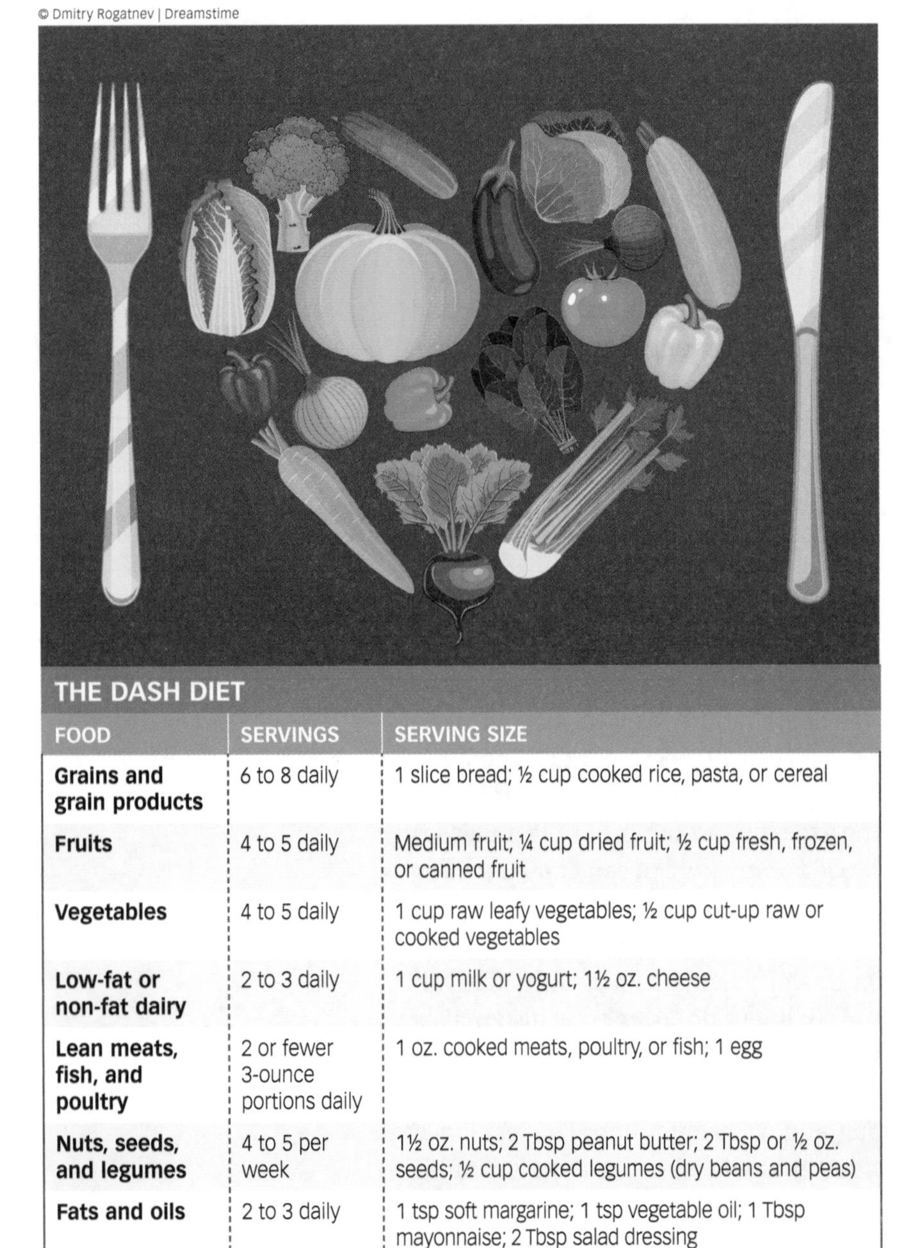

THE DASH DIET

FOOD	SERVINGS	SERVING SIZE
Grains and grain products	6 to 8 daily	1 slice bread; ½ cup cooked rice, pasta, or cereal
Fruits	4 to 5 daily	Medium fruit; ¼ cup dried fruit; ½ cup fresh, frozen, or canned fruit
Vegetables	4 to 5 daily	1 cup raw leafy vegetables; ½ cup cut-up raw or cooked vegetables
Low-fat or non-fat dairy	2 to 3 daily	1 cup milk or yogurt; 1½ oz. cheese
Lean meats, fish, and poultry	2 or fewer 3-ounce portions daily	1 oz. cooked meats, poultry, or fish; 1 egg
Nuts, seeds, and legumes	4 to 5 per week	1½ oz. nuts; 2 Tbsp peanut butter; 2 Tbsp or ½ oz. seeds; ½ cup cooked legumes (dry beans and peas)
Fats and oils	2 to 3 daily	1 tsp soft margarine; 1 tsp vegetable oil; 1 Tbsp mayonnaise; 2 Tbsp salad dressing
Sweets and added sugars	5 or less per week	1 Tbsp sugar; 1 Tbsp jelly or jam; ½ cup sorbet or gelatin

physician about whether you can use salt substitutes.

To lower your sodium intake:

- Reduce salt use gradually to allow your taste buds to adjust.
- Use herbs and spices rather than salt to flavor your food, and consider using onion, garlic, lemon juice, and vinegar for added flavor.
- When you dine out, ask your server to make sure that salt, monosodium glutamate (MSG, a flavor enhancer commonly used in Chinese food), and seasoned salt are omitted.

Watch for Other Sources of Sodium

Many over-the-counter products contain sodium, including medications for colds, headaches, upset stomach, and other ailments; vitamins and mineral supplements; food supplements; and nutraceuticals (food-derived products that may have a medicinal effect). Sodium compounds found in such products include sodium ascorbate, sodium bicarbonate, sodium phosphate, sodium biphosphate, sodium citrate, sodium fluoride, sodium saccharin, and sodium salicylate. If you see the word "sodium" anywhere on the label, look for a comparable product with no sodium or less sodium. If no substitute is available, it's advisable to avoid the product altogether.

Limit Your Fluid Intake

Too much fluid will contribute to congestion and swelling, increasing your heart's workload. Your physician will tell you whether you need to restrict fluids—if so, follow your fluid-management guidelines carefully.

As a general rule, fluid intake should be limited to less than eight cups per day (including coffee and tea). This is equivalent to about two liters, two quarts, or one-half gallon. Keep a daily record of your fluid intake until you feel comfortable with your restrictions and can accurately determine how much fluid you are consuming. It helps to learn

Foods Naturally Low in Sodium

Finding foods that are compatible with a low-sodium diet can be challenging, but plenty are available. Here are some suggestions:

Basic Foods

- Lean meat (fresh chicken, turkey, pork, or roast beef)
- Fresh or frozen fish (not breaded)
- Fresh vegetables and frozen vegetables without added sauce
- Bread, rolls, and bagels
- Dried beans and legumes
- Plain rice or pasta
- Low-sodium soup, broth, or bouillon
- Eggs
- Fat-free or low-fat milk and yogurt
- Low- or reduced-sodium cheese
- Fresh fruits and frozen or dried fruit

Sweets and Snacks

- Sherbet, sorbet, Italian ice, and Popsicles
- Unsalted nuts and seeds
- Low-sodium potato chips, pretzels, and popcorn

Condiments, Seasonings, Fats, and Oils

- Vegetable oils
- Unsalted butter or margarine
- Ginger
- Low-sodium ketchup and mustard
- Low-sodium salad dressing
- Herbs, spices, or salt-free seasoning blends
- Vinegar

High-Sodium Foods to Avoid

Always check the label on these foods for the amount of sodium they contain:

- Snack foods, including dips
- Boxed cereals
- Processed foods, including frozen foods
- Canned foods, such as stews, casseroles, and beans
- Canned or dry soups
- Vegetable juice drinks
- Frozen or boxed mixes of potatoes, rice, and pasta
- Commercial baking mixes
- Condiments, such as soy sauce, relish, catsup, and mustard

These foods are almost always high in sodium:

- Luncheon meats
- Smoked, cured, salted, and canned meats
- Bacon, ham, corned beef, sausage, and hot dogs
- "Fast food"
- TV dinners
- Processed cheeses
- Gatorade and similar drinks
- Bottled salad dressing
- Bottled spaghetti sauce
- Soy sauce
- Pickles and olives
- Canned pork and beans, and sauerkraut
- Bottled, canned, and dry marinades, gravies and sauces (such as steak and barbecue sauces)
- Meat tenderizers, flavor enhancers (such as MSG), and seasoned salts

Sodium Content of Some Common Foods

FOOD	SERVING SIZE	MILLIGRAMS SODIUM
MEAT, POULTRY, FISH, SHELLFISH		
Fresh meat	3 oz. cooked	90+
Raw shellfish	3 oz.	126-711
Tuna, canned	3 oz.	287-375
Lean ham	3 oz.	1,289
Deli meats	1 oz. slice	178-426
VEGETABLES		
Vegetables, canned or frozen (without sauce)	½ cup	55-480
Tomato juice, canned	¾ cup	660
DAIRY PRODUCTS		
Whole milk	1 cup	120
Skim or 1 percent milk	1 cup	125
Buttermilk (salt added)	1 cup	260
Swiss cheese	1 oz.	75
Cheddar cheese	1 oz.	175
Low-fat cheese	1 oz.	150
Cottage cheese (regular)	½ cup	455
BREADS, CEREALS, RICE, PASTA		
Bread	1 slice	110-175
English muffin	½	130
Ready-to-eat cereal	¾-1 cup	4-322
Cooked cereal (unsalted)	½ cup	5+
Instant cooked cereal	1 packet	120-377
CONVENIENCE FOODS		
Spaghetti sauce	½ cup	370-1,513
Canned soup	1 cup	600-1,300
Frozen entrees	8 oz.	564-1,594
FAST FOODS		
Fast-food breakfast sandwich		804-1,540
Fast-food sandwich		513-2,320
Fast-food submarine sandwich		310-1,900
Pizza slice		267-382
Fries or onion rings		135-1,540

the fluid volumes (cups, fluid ounces, or liters) in a serving of your favorite foods. Keep in mind that ice is a fluid, and count ice and foods that are considered fluids (like soup, pudding, frozen yogurt, applesauce, and all fruits, particularly citrus) against your daily fluid allowance.

Instead of drinking a beverage, quench your thirst by nibbling on frozen grapes or strawberries, or by eating sugarless hard candy or chewing sugarless gum. Covering your lips with lip balm also may help. And keep in mind that milk and ice cream products increase thirst.

Stay Alert for Signs of Fluid Retention. Although the most obvious sign of fluid retention is weight gain, there may be other clues:

- Your belt seems tighter.
- Your belly appears more swollen.
- Your clothes don't fit as well.
- Your feet and ankles swell.
- Your shoes become tight.
- Your shoelaces seem shorter.
- You are short of breath.
- You cough, especially when you are laying down.
- You wake at night because of difficulty breathing.
- You feel full after eating only a small amount of food.

Weigh yourself every day at the same time, using the same scale and wearing clothing of similar weight (or none). Record your weight daily in a diary or on a calendar.

If you have symptoms of congestion—especially if you feel more fatigued than usual or have shortness of breath along with weight gain—call your doctor. Otherwise, for two days try eliminating 500 mg of sodium from your diet and decreasing your fluid intake by one-and-a-half cups (12 oz). If your swelling and weight do not go down after two days, call your doctor. Your medications may need to be adjusted.

To keep track of your daily sodium and fluid intake, see the Sodium and Fluid Intake Record Form at the end of this Special Report.

Avoid Alcohol

Alcohol weakens the heart's pumping ability and may make you more likely to develop abnormal heart rhythms. Limiting your alcohol consumption to no more than one drink daily (or not drinking at all) is recommended. One drink means 12 ounces of beer, four to five ounces of wine, or one ounce of 80-proof liquor. If your doctor tells you that you can safely have one drink a day, remember to count it against your total daily fluid allowance.

Get Active and Exercise Regularly

Many people with heart failure are surprised to hear that exercise is beneficial, because they think that exerting themselves is the last thing they should do. However, exercise can improve quality of life and reduce heart failure symptoms and hospital readmissions. It may even ward off death from heart failure or other heart causes.

Even minimal exercise produces modest reductions in heart failure risk, but the more exercise you get, the lower your risk will drop. When you are active, you may have more energy, be less irritable, sleep better, and be better able to keep your weight under control.

Inactivity can cause your physical condition to deteriorate, because your muscles will lose their ability to function and your bones will weaken. When this happens, the heart must pump more blood to the muscles to produce the necessary energy, which in turn stresses the heart. Exercise also improves blood flow to the arms and legs. However, you should not start an exercise program without asking your cardiologist how much exercise you can do each day and what kind of activities are right for you. Your efforts should match your capacity, and as your capacity improves, so can your effort.

Even if you can't exercise on your own, you can participate in cardiac rehabilitation. These programs are monitored and adjusted to help you exercise safely. Active participation in a cardiac rehabilitation program is associated with better outcomes in heart failure patients. Medicare and many insurance companies now pay for cardiac rehabilitation. If your doctor does not refer you to a program, request a referral.

If the thought of a formal exercise program overwhelms you, keep in mind that any exercise is better than no exercise at all, and exercise does not have to be intense to be beneficial. Healthy choices include walking, bicycling, or practicing tai chi, an ancient Chinese martial art that combines slow, flowing movement and meditation.

An exercise test can help determine your exercise capacity, or how much exercise you can do. Based on the test results, an exercise physiologist will prepare an individual exercise prescription. That prescription initially may be for as little as five to 10 minutes on a stationary bicycle or walking a few times a week at a relatively slow pace. The intensity and duration of exercise will be gradually increased.

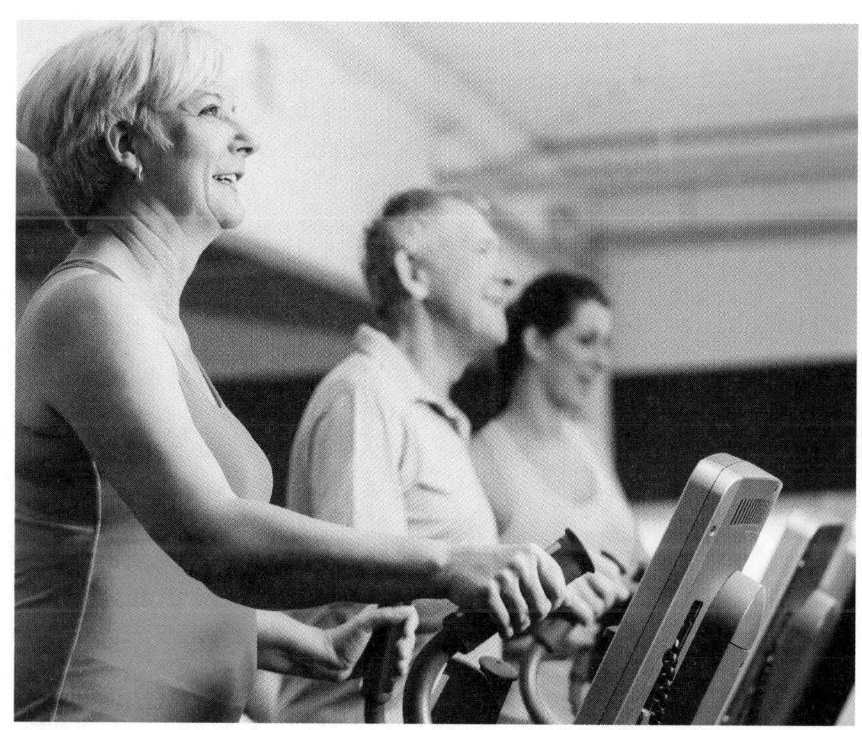

Exercise can improve quality of life for people with heart failure.

Lose Excess Weight

Excess weight is a major risk factor for heart failure. According to the National Center for Health Statistics, 71.6 percent of U.S. adults are overweight or obese. If you fall into one of these two categories, or your doctor has recommended that you lose weight, make an effort to shed the excess pounds. Preparing fresh foods—or purchasing prepared meals that are low in sodium and contain the right balance of fat, protein, and carbohydrates for someone with heart disease—will help you lose weight.

Although it may be tempting to try "fad" diets, Cleveland Clinic cardiologists do not recommend these. Many diets promote drinking large quantities of water, which can be detrimental in heart failure. You may lose weight rapidly on certain popular diets, but their limited choice of foods makes them difficult to follow for very long, and 90 percent of people regain the lost weight after they stop the diet. The Ornish diet is safe for people with heart failure, but it is highly restrictive. The South Beach Diet is not considered a fad diet, because it is scientifically sound. You also may find it easier to follow than the Ornish diet. It may be helpful to consult with a registered, licensed dietitian (RD, LD) to plan a healthful diet.

If you are finding it difficult to lose weight, discuss with your doctor whether bariatric surgery might be an option for you. A 2018 Cleveland Clinic study found that weight-loss surgery had a significant protective effect on survival. People with heart failure who had undergone weight-loss surgery at any time had nearly half the risk of in-hospital death as those who had never had the surgery. This indicates that in addition to promoting weight loss, bariatric surgery benefits the heart in other ways.

Get Sufficient Rest

Ensuring that you get enough rest may not be difficult, because heart failure causes fatigue. You may have to adjust your work schedule or activities to accommodate the extra rest time. Plan activities ahead of time, and do not schedule too many in one day. Also, do not push, pull, or lift heavy objects that require you to strain or quickly tire you.

Accept that on some days you may have more energy, but if you are more active on one day, you may feel more tired the next. When you wear out, simply stop and rest. It's okay to nap, but try not to nap too often or too long, or you may not be able to sleep well at night. It is important to sleep as well as possible. Good sleep practices include:

- Avoiding caffeine and alcohol before bedtime.
- Avoiding strenuous activity just before bedtime.
- Reserving your bed for sleeping, not for watching television, reading, or eating.
- Developing specific bedtime rituals and sticking to them.
- Going to bed and getting up at the same time every day.
- Aiming for seven to eight hours of sleep every night.
- Asking your doctor to adjust your medications so that you can get uninterrupted sleep.
- If you still have difficulty sleeping, ask your doctor if a sleep medication would help you drift off at night.

Take Care of Your Mental Health

High levels of stress can be detrimental to your physical and emotional health. Recognizing stress and learning how to manage it can improve your quality of life and benefit your heart. About half of people with heart failure experience depression. In people with heart failure, mild depression increases the risk of death by 60 percent and moderate-to-severe depression quadruples the risk. Signs of depression include persistent feelings of sadness, mood swings, and lack of pleasure in things you used to enjoy. If you think you may be depressed, talk with your doctor. Medications and therapies can help you restore a healthier outlook and may even save your life.

Different stress-management techniques work for different people. Often,

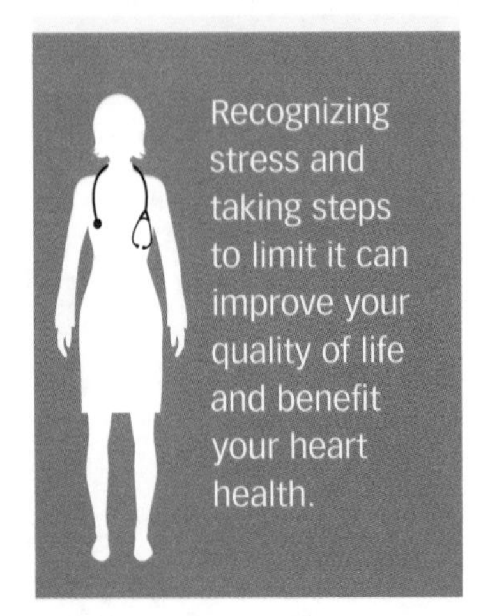

a combination of methods proves most useful. Some things you can do to reduce stress include:

- Follow an exercise program and remain as active as possible.
- Perform relaxation exercises or yoga to calm the body and mind.
- Try prayer, meditation, or tai chi.
- Join a support group—talking to others can help.
- Seek one-on-one counseling for guided support.
- Enjoy social activities and time spent with friends.

Protect Your General Health

Minor illnesses that most people shrug off can seriously affect people with heart failure. You also may be laid low by hot weather and overexertion. Follow these tips to stay safe:

- Call your doctor if you have symptoms of a respiratory infection (sore throat, runny nose, persistent cough, fever, and general aches and pains).
- Avoid contact with anyone who has a cold, the flu, or bronchitis.
- Get a flu shot every year. The benefits of flu shots far outweigh the risks.
- Consider getting the Pneumovax pneumonia vaccination. This usually is given only once, with a booster every five years.
- Avoid temperature extremes, and stay indoors when it is very hot or very cold outside. High humidity levels may cause you to become fatigued more easily.
- Avoid lifting or pushing heavy objects or doing strenuous chores, such as raking, mowing, shoveling, or scrubbing. If you find household chores exhausting, ask for help or hire someone.
- If you become fatigued or experience shortness of breath during any activity, slow down, or stop and rest. Be sure to tell your doctor about it. You may need changes in your medications, diet, or fluid consumption.
- If you develop a rapid or irregular heartbeat or palpitations, check your pulse. If your heart rate is higher than 120 beats per minute, call your doctor or go to the emergency department.
- If you feel faint or lose consciousness, your family or friends should call 911. It may indicate a life-threatening arrhythmia or low blood pressure (hypotension). Make sure the incident is reported to your cardiologist, and discuss it with your doctor as soon as you are able.
- If you have shortness of breath at night, try sleeping in a recliner chair, or use more pillows or a supportive wedge cushion to elevate your upper body.
- Thoughtfully consider the need for elective surgery before you proceed with this (see "Outpatient Surgery Increases Risk").

Lifestyle Modifications May Not Be Enough

Lifestyle modifications often help alleviate symptoms, but they cannot cure or reverse heart failure. At some point, you will need medications. Together, lifestyle adjustments and medications are far more effective than either approach alone.

NEW FINDING

Outpatient Surgery Increases Risk

Ambulatory surgery is generally considered low risk. However, it may be somewhat riskier than expected for heart failure patients. A study of more than 355,000 people in a Veterans' Affairs Surgical Quality Improvement database revealed that those with heart failure had a higher 90-day mortality rate than those without heart failure. The risk was progressively higher as heart function declined. For your own protection, discuss plans for any type of outpatient operation with your cardiologist, so that you will be closely monitored.

JAMA Surgery, July 2019

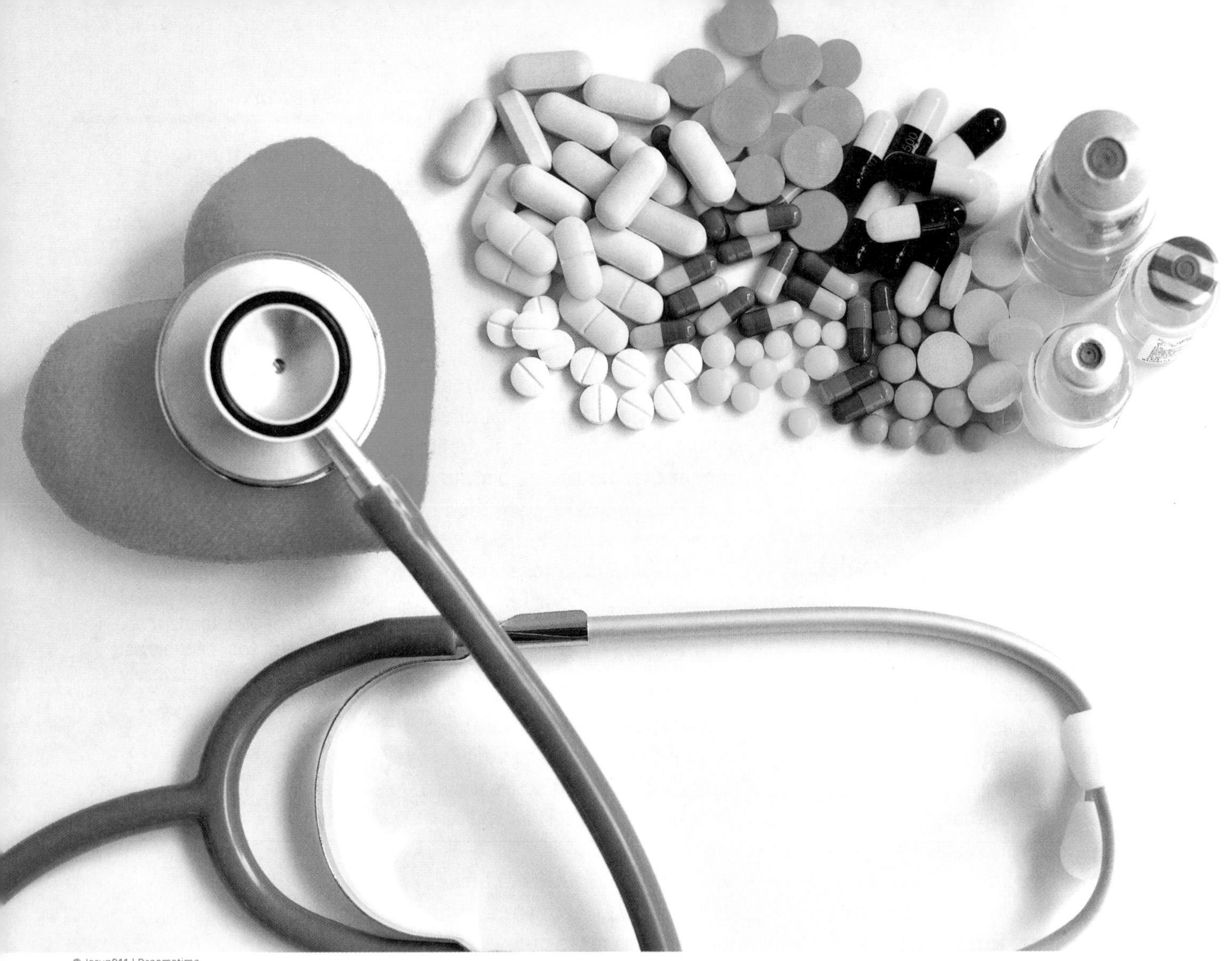

© Jarun011 | Dreamstime

A range of effective medications is available to treat heart failure.

7 Medical Treatments for Heart Failure

In recent years, dramatic developments in drug therapy for heart failure have occurred. Physicians now can choose from a variety of medications to individualize heart failure care. The most effective medication and dosage for each person varies depending on the severity of their heart failure and coexisting conditions. Race also may play a role in some treatment decisions, as certain medications work differently in different ethnic groups.

In the past, standard medical therapy for heart failure consisted of three main classes of drugs: digoxin (Digox, Digitek), which increases the heart's pumping ability; a diuretic to eliminate excess fluid; and an angiotensin-converting enzyme (ACE) inhibitor to increase blood flow. Guidelines now recommend that in addition to a diuretic plus ACE inhibitor or angiotensin receptor blocker (ARB), patients be started on a beta-blocker and a renin-angiotensin antagonist within one month of being diagnosed with heart failure. If they remain symptomatic, an aldosterone antagonist or hydralazine/nitrate should be added.

As heart failure worsens, treatment becomes more complex, and surgery may be advised.

Treatment Strategies

The following is a guideline of treatment strategies for each stage of heart failure, based on the classification system used by the American College of Cardiology (ACC) and the American Heart Association (AHA):

Stage A

This stage includes people who don't have heart failure symptoms but are considered to be at high risk of developing heart failure. Stage A treatment focuses on eliminating risk factors through lifestyle modifications, such as weight loss, exercise, and avoidance of tobacco, illicit drugs, and excessive alcohol. Patients with diabetes and/or confirmed coronary artery disease should be prescribed ACE inhibitors or ARBs, statins (cholesterol-lowering drugs), and/or low-dose aspirin.

Stage B

People in this group have no apparent symptoms of heart failure, but have confirmed structural heart disease. Many have had a heart attack, others have cardiomyopathy or valve disease. People at stage B should follow the lifestyle modifications and take the medications listed for stage A. Most also should take an ACE inhibitor or ARB, and a beta-blocker.

Stage C

This group includes people who have structural heart disease and symptoms of heart failure, such as shortness of breath, fatigue, and reduced exercise tolerance. In addition to all measures appropriate for stages A and B, these individuals should restrict their salt intake, use a diuretic, and take an ACE inhibitor or an ARB, plus a beta-blocker. In some, digoxin may be recommended. An aldosterone antagonist may be prescribed for left ventricular (LV) dysfunction and mild-to-severe heart failure symptoms or after a heart attack.

In some cases, surgical intervention may be considered for people whose heart failure has progressed to stage C (see Chapter 8). An implantable cardioverter defibrillator is recommended for the majority of people with a left ventricular ejection fraction of less than 35 percent and symptoms of heart failure. Some may be eligible for cardiac resynchronization therapy (see Chapter 8).

Stage D

Patients who have progressed to stage D are severely ill and require special medical and/or surgical intervention. Intravenous diuretics and vasodilators may be appropriate for hospitalized patients, and some may be considered for a heart transplant, ventricular assist device, and/or investigational surgery or drugs (see Chapter 8). End-stage patients who are not eligible for any of these extraordinary procedures may be referred for hospice care.

Medications Commonly Used in the Treatment of Heart Failure

TYPE OF DRUG	WHAT IT DOES
Aldosterone blocker	Blocks the harmful effects of the hormone aldosterone in patients with heart failure.
Angiotensin-converting enzyme (ACE) inhibitor	Dilates blood vessels to reduce blood pressure, improves the heart's output of blood, and increases blood flow to the kidneys. ACE inhibitors also block the production of angiotensin II.
Angiotensin receptor blocker (ARB)	ARBs have the same effects as ACE inhibitors.
Angiotensin receptor/neprilysin inhibitor (ARNI)	Relaxes blood vessels and eliminates excess fluid and sodium.
Anti-arrhythmic agent	Controls the heart's rhythm and prevents the generation of an irregular rhythm.
Anticoagulant and antiplatelet agent	Prevents the formation of potentially harmful blood clots, especially in heart failure patients with atrial fibrillation.
Beta-blocker	Slows the heart rate and reduces blood pressure. By blocking the "beta receptors" of the heart, it also blocks the detrimental action of excess norepinephrine (noradrenaline) on the heart muscle.
Digoxin	Improves the heart's pumping ability and lowers abnormally high levels of neurohormones that aggravate heart failure.
Diuretic	Removes extra fluid from the tissues and bloodstream, lessens edema (swelling), and makes breathing easier.
Hydralazine/nitrate	Dilates (opens) the arteries and veins.
Inotropic agent	Improves the heart's pumping function and raises blood pressure in patients with cardiogenic shock or low cardiac output.
Nesiritide	Administered intravenously to reduce high pressures within the heart and lungs and to improve acute decompensated heart failure symptoms.
Potassium and magnesium	Replace salts lost with increased urination in patients who take certain diuretics.
Vasodilator	Dilates (opens) the arteries and veins.

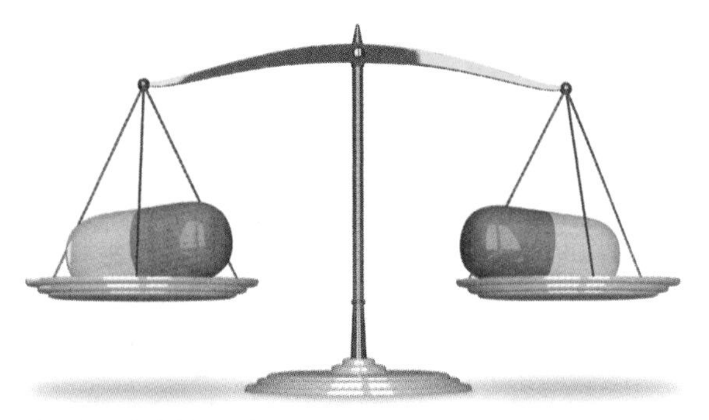

© Dmitryguzhanin | Dreamstime

It is vital to balance heart failure medications so that side effects do not occur.

Balancing Medications

Balancing medications in heart failure is a difficult job. Between 17 and 22 percent of patients with mildly symptomatic heart failure develop anemia due to iron deficiency or the inability of their kidneys to produce enough of the hormone erythropoietin, which plays a key role in the production of red blood cells. As heart failure progresses, anemia becomes more common, affecting up to 70 percent of people with New York Heart Association (NYHA) class IV heart failure (see Chapter 5). The condition, which is associated with poor survival, can be caused or aggravated by sodium and water retention, kidney disease, or other processes associated with heart failure.

When appropriate, treatment with erythropoietic agents may help. However, these drugs may increase the risk of blood clots and are tricky to administer. They also are expensive. In people who are iron-deficient, oral or intravenous iron supplementation can boost hemoglobin, the oxygen-carrying protein found in red blood cells. Iron-replacement therapy has been shown to improve exercise tolerance, NYHA class, and quality of life.

Early Warning Devices

Because it often is difficult to balance medications to eliminate the maximum amount of sodium and water without upsetting the body's chemistry, doctors are optimistic about the value of "early warning" devices in heart failure treatment. These implantable devices are designed to sense changes in intracardiac pressures that signal the beginnings of excess fluid buildup in the heart and lungs. The CardioMEMS device has proven to be particularly successful. It enables a physician to adjust medications to prevent pulmonary edema and its consequences, ultimately helping heart failure patients feel better and reducing crises that require hospitalization. In a 2017 study of Medicare enrollees, the CardioMEMS device reduced hospitalizations by 45 percent in the six months after the device was implanted, saving $13,000 per patient per year. The U.S. Food and Drug Administration (FDA) approved the device in 2014 for people with NYHA class III heart failure who have been hospitalized for heart failure within the past year.

ACE Inhibitors Used in Heart Failure

DRUG	INITIAL DOSE	TARGET DOSE AND FREQUENCY
Captopril (Capoten)	6.25 mg	50 mg three times daily
Enalapril (Vasotec)	2.5 mg	20 mg twice daily
Fosinopril (Monopril)	10 mg	40 mg daily
Lisinopril (Prinivil, Zestril)	5 mg	20-40 mg daily
Quinapril (Accupril)	10 mg	20 mg twice daily
Ramipril (Altace)	1.25 mg	10 mg daily

Common Heart Failure Medications

The following is a detailed overview of the drugs that have proven beneficial for people with heart failure.

ACE Inhibitors

Until ACE inhibitors were developed, a diagnosis of heart failure—even mild heart failure—was associated with a short life expectancy. ACE inhibitors changed that picture significantly and are a major contributor in the improved prognosis for heart failure patients who receive treatment early in the course of the condition.

ACE inhibitors work by dilating blood vessels, which allows blood to flow more easily. When the kidneys release renin, a cascade of reactions takes place that ultimately generates a hormone called angiotensin II, which constricts small arteries and raises blood pressure. ACE inhibitors block the key enzyme in this cascade. When angiotensin II production drops, arteries relax and dilate, and blood pressure drops.

Numerous clinical trials have shown that ACE inhibitors decrease the incidence of sudden death, heart attack, and stroke, improve quality of life, and enhance blood flow to the kidneys, thereby improving sodium excretion. They also increase exercise tolerance and prevent—sometimes reverse—ventricular remodeling. In people with the earliest stage of heart failure, ACE inhibitors can prevent heart attack and stroke.

ACC/AHA guidelines recommend ACE inhibitors for anyone at increased risk of heart failure due to hypertension, diabetes, or atherosclerosis. Those guidelines also call for ACE inhibitor use in all patients with evidence of structural heart disease (with or without symptoms) and in patients with the most severe heart failure. People with high potassium levels (hyperkalemia), a history of angioedema (swelling of the face and throat), and some patients with impaired kidney function should not take ACE inhibitors.

ACE Inhibitor Side Effects. The maximum benefit of ACE inhibitors is seen at the recommended doses. However, therapy usually is started at a lower dose to reduce side effects. Once a dose is well tolerated, it is increased, and the process is repeated. It may take up to three months for the full benefit of an ACE inhibitor to be realized.

A common side effect of ACE inhibitors is a dry cough. Although this can be annoying, most people will tolerate it in exchange for the drug's proven benefits. Because heart failure itself can cause a cough, the ACE inhibitor is not always to blame. Nevertheless, if the cough is annoying, switching to an angiotensin II receptor blocker (ARB) may be appropriate. Other possible side effects of ACE inhibitors include dizziness and an abnormal sense of taste. If ACE inhibitors make you dizzy, avoid caffeine, alcohol, and overeating. A small number of people are allergic to ACE inhibitors and may experience swelling of the face or other parts of the body (angioedema) due to the drugs.

Angiotensin II Receptor Blockers Used in Heart Failure

DRUG	INITIAL DOSE	TARGET DOSE AND FREQUENCY
Candesartan (Atacand)	4 mg	32 mg daily
Valsartan (Diovan)	40 mg	160 mg twice daily

ARBs

Like ACE inhibitors, ARBs also interfere with the renin-angiotensin-aldosterone system. However, instead of blocking the formation of angiotensin II—as ACE inhibitors do—they block the effect of angiotensin II on organs and tissues. ARBs typically do not cause a cough.

Two ARBs—valsartan (Diovan) and candesartan (Atacand)—have been approved by the FDA for use in people with heart failure. Several other ARBs also are commonly used in heart failure, although they are not FDA-approved for this purpose. The most popular one is losartan (Cozaar). ARBs are primarily used in patients with systolic heart failure. At this time Cleveland Clinic cardiologists recommend patients take only branded ARBs (see "FDA Recalls Generic ARBs").

If you have heart failure with a low ejection fraction and cannot tolerate ACE inhibitors, taking candesartan in addition to other heart failure medications is better than not taking an ARB. If you are able to tolerate ACE inhibitors, adding the ARB candesartan may provide additional protection from death or hospitalization.

ARB Side Effects. ARBs are generally well tolerated but can cause dizziness, headache, and cough, although the latter is

NEW FINDING

FDA Recalls Generic ARBs

In July 2018, the U.S. Food and Drug Administration (FDA) found N-nitrosodimethylamine (NDMA), a potential carcinogen used in rocket fuel, in generic versions of the angiotensin receptor blocker (ARB) valsartan (Diovan) made in India. The FDA recalled the drug, and in successive months recalled generic versions of the ARBs losartan (Cozaar) and irbesartan (Avapro) when a second related carcinogen (NDEA) was discovered. A third related carcinogen (NMBA) was found in early 2019. Most of the products were manufactured in India and China by different companies, some for American-based pharmaceutical companies. Whether these chemicals are actually harmful at the levels found in the drugs is unknown (the FDA claims they are not). However, until the cause of the contamination is discovered and contained, it may be wise to request the brand-name version of your ARB, avoid generic ARBs made outside the United States, or ask your doctor if you can switch to an angiotensin-converting enzyme inhibitor (ACE inhibitor).

FDA Drug Recalls, May 23, 2019

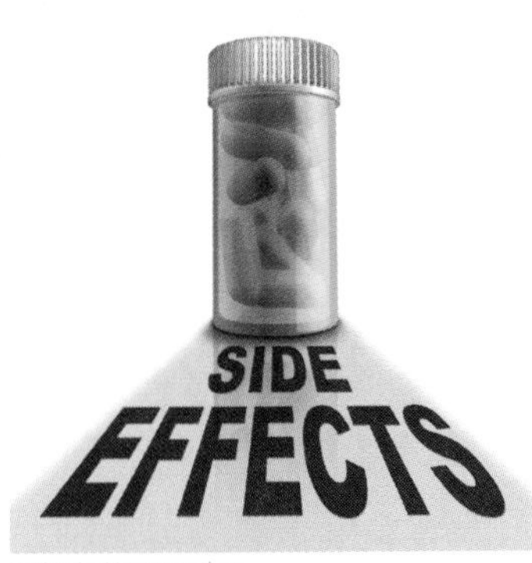

© Skypixel | Dreamstime

It is vital that you report any possible medication side effects to your doctor.

much less likely than with ACE inhibitors. Most physicians start heart failure patients on a diuretic plus an ACE inhibitor, and only switch to an ARB if the ACE inhibitor is not tolerated.

ARNIs

Cardiologists consider angiotensin receptor/neprilysin inhibitors (ARNIs) to be one of the most exciting developments in heart failure in decades. These drugs are very effective at relaxing blood vessels and eliminating excess fluid and sodium.

In clinical trials, the first drug in this class, sacubitril/valsartan (Entresto) showed dramatic ability to reduce deaths and hospitalizations in people with heart failure. Its benefits were so striking that the FDA expedited approval of the drug. It has since been shown to boost heart failure patients' quality of life in many ways, particularly by increasing the ability to do daily chores and enjoy sexual relationships.

ARNIs are now recommended as a replacement for ACE inhibitors and ARBs in people with NYHA II and III heart failure and an ejection fraction of less than 35 percent, to further lower hospitalizations and mortality.

ARNI Side Effects. ARNIs should not be taken with ACE inhibitors or ARBS. If you switch to an ARNI from either of these drugs, you will likely need a period of about 36 hours between stopping the old drug and taking the ARNI. Possible side effects from ARNIs include low blood pressure (hypotension), elevated potassium levels, dizziness, and cough.

Beta-Blockers Used in Heart Failure

DRUG	INITIAL DOSE	TARGET DOSE AND FREQUENCY
Carvedilol (Coreg)	3.125 mg	25-50 mg twice daily
Metoprolol succinate (Toprol XL)	12.5-25 mg	200 mg daily
Bisoprolol (Zebata)	1.25-2.5 mg	10 mg daily

Beta-Blockers

People with heart failure and high levels of norepinephrine in their blood have an increased risk of death. Beta-blockers modulate the activity of the sympathetic nervous system that produces norepinephrine.

Adding beta-blockers to other heart failure drugs improves survival by as much as 34 percent. That's why guidelines recommend that heart failure patients take beta-blockers in addition to diuretics and ACE inhibitors.

In addition to increasing survival, beta-blockers slow heart failure progression, improve NYHA functional class, and reduce the risk of heart arrhythmias and hospitalization. They also may prevent many of the harmful effects of ventricular remodeling by increasing ejection fraction and decreasing the size of the heart. These biologic effects appear to reverse remodeling. Beta-blockers also lessen the symptoms of heart failure, thus helping people with the condition feel better.

ACC/AHA heart failure guidelines recommend beta-blockers for people with left ventricular systolic dysfunction but no symptoms, those with stable NYHA class II-IV heart failure, and all patients who have had a heart attack, regardless of whether they have heart failure. The Joint Commission, an independent body that accredits and certifies health-care organizations, requires that heart failure patients be given a prescription for beta-blockers when they are discharged from the hospital.

Beta-Blocker Side Effects. Finding the proper dose of a beta-blocker is extremely important, because the drug can slow the heart rate or lower blood pressure, further limiting the heart's ability to pump efficiently. Different beta-blockers come in a variety of strengths and are taken once or twice a day. The dose of a beta-blocker may be doubled every two weeks until the maximum tolerated dose is reached.

The most common side effects of beta-blockers are dizziness, slow heartbeat (bradycardia), shortness of breath, and fatigue. These effects usually can be managed by adjusting the dose. However, it is important that you never adjust the dose on your own. Other side effects may include cold hands and feet, headache, difficulty sleeping, wheezing, rash, swelling of the feet and legs, and sudden weight gain.

People with acutely decompensated heart failure (a sudden worsening of heart failure symptoms) should not use beta-blockers. Those with very severe diabetes, asthma, or peripheral vascular disease may not be able to tolerate beta-blockers. Your cardiologist may decide to prescribe beta-blockers in these situations, but you will need to be carefully monitored.

When a symptomatic heart failure patient cannot take beta-blockers or tolerate the recommended dose, ivabradine (Corlanor) may be used instead. Ivabradine slows the heart rate like beta-blockers do, enabling it to pump more effectively.

Diuretics

Diuretics (also known as water pills) cause the kidneys to excrete more water and sodium. They are used to eliminate excess fluid and decrease swelling.

The three main types of diuretic—thiazide, loop, and potassium-sparing—work differently. Thiazide diuretics are most commonly used to treat high blood pressure, while the more powerful loop diuretics often are used in kidney and heart failure. Potassium-sparing diuretics are weaker and typically are combined with thiazide or loop diuretics to prevent the potassium loss that occurs with diuretic use.

Heart failure specialists prescribe diuretics for approximately 90 percent of patients and strive to use the lowest effective dose. You may be allowed to adjust your own diuretics based on your symptoms, following specific instructions from your doctor. You will monitor your weight daily, and if you gain more than three pounds above your normal baseline weight, you may increase the diuretic dose as instructed.

Some people with mild or moderate heart failure who take an ACE inhibitor and beta-blocker do not need to take a daily diuretic. However, as heart failure becomes more severe, diuretic requirements typically increase. Not complying with your sodium and fluid restrictions also will lead to greater fluid retention and a heavier reliance on diuretics.

Diuretic Side Effects. The diuretic your doctor prescribes will depend on your individual needs, and you may need to take a combination of drugs.

Most heart failure patients are started on a loop diuretic such as furosemide (Lasix), torsemide (Demadex), or bumetanide (Bumex). If a stronger diuretic effect is needed, a combination of loop and thiazide diuretics is

Diuretics Used in Heart Failure

DRUG	INITIAL DOSE	TARGET DOSE AND FREQUENCY
THIAZIDE DIURETICS		
Hydrochlorothiazide (Hydrodiuril)	25 mg	50 mg
Chlorthalidone (Hygroton)	25 mg	50 mg
Indapamide (generic only)	2.5 mg twice daily	5 mg
Metolazone (Zaroxolyn)	2.5 mg	10 mg
LOOP DIURETICS		
Furosemide (Lasix)	10-40 mg	240 mg twice daily
Torsemide (Demadex)	10 mg	200 mg
Bumetanide (Bumex)	0.5-1.0 mg	10 mg
POTASSIUM-SPARING DIURETICS		
Spironolactone (Aldactone)	25 mg	50 mg twice daily
Triamterene (Dyrenium)	50 mg	100 mg twice daily
Amiloride (Midamor)	5 mg	20 mg
Eplerenone (Inspira)	25 mg	50 mg

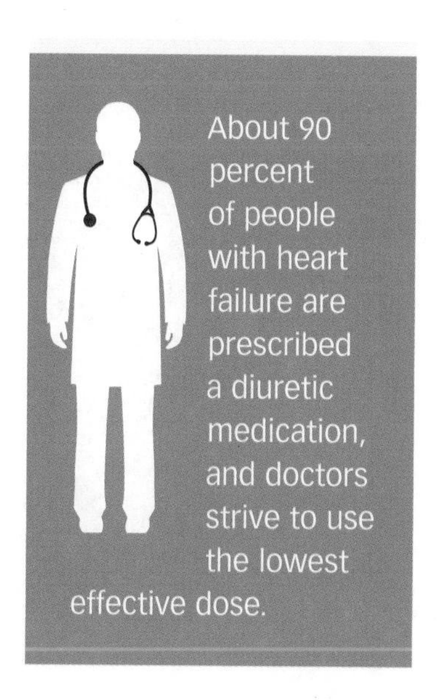

given. Spironolactone (Aldactone) is a potassium-sparing diuretic and neurohormonal modulator that improves survival in people with severe heart failure when it is added to therapy with an ACE inhibitor, beta-blocker, digoxin, and diuretics.

Diuretic doses are based on the severity of heart failure, as well as on diet, salt and fluid intake, activity level, and kidney function. Doses are adjusted as needed to relieve swelling and congestion. High doses can cause fluid and electrolyte imbalances from loss of sodium and water. Loss of too much sodium can cause low blood pressure, dehydration, and worsening kidney function. Overly aggressive use of diuretics also can cause imbalances in other minerals and electrolytes in the body, including potassium, magnesium, calcium, and chloride. Elderly or debilitated individuals are more susceptible to these adverse effects than younger heart failure patients.

People with acute decompensated heart failure typically require large doses of diuretics delivered intravenously to drain the extra fluid from their bodies. However, they often stop responding to conventional diuretics. Ularitide, a synthetic natriuretic peptide, was developed as an alternative treatment for this patient population. In the TRUE-AHF trial, the drug relieved congestion and made people feel better within 48 hours, but had no effect on long-term outcomes.

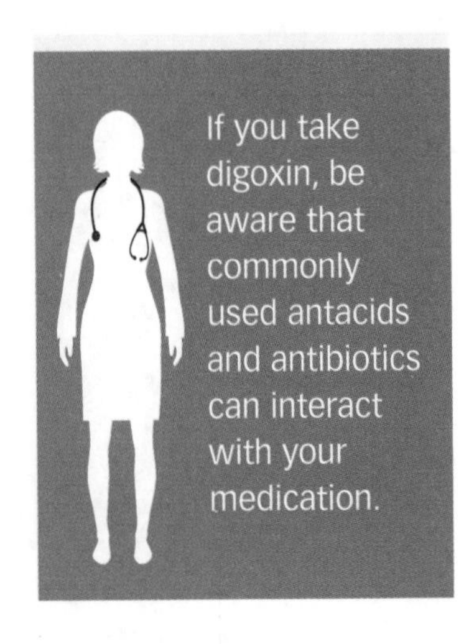

If you take diuretics, it is important to keep your blood potassium level normal to prevent abnormal heart rhythms. Potassium-sparing diuretics raise blood potassium levels. Thiazide and loop diuretics lower blood potassium levels. Either way, severe potassium imbalances produce the same symptoms: weakness, numbness, confusion, and heaviness in the legs. If you take a thiazide or a loop diuretic and are not on a potassium-sparing diuretic, it is important to eat potassium-rich foods such as baked potatoes, dried fruit, bananas, white beans, cantaloupe, and spinach. You also may need a potassium supplement. However, you should never take a potassium supplement or a salt substitute containing potassium unless advised to do so by your doctor, no matter which type of diuretic you are taking.

A few people who use diuretics find that they develop a rash. The drugs also may increase your sensitivity to the sun (research has linked thiazide diuretics to a greater risk of skin cancer). Protect yourself by staying out of the sun when it is at its strongest (between 10 a.m. and 4 p.m.) and wearing plenty of factor 30 or higher sunscreen if you spend time outdoors in sunny weather. Another common effect of diuretic use is dry mouth. If this happens to you, use sugar-free hard candy to stimulate the flow of saliva. People who take diuretics also are more susceptible to attacks of gout, a type of arthritis that causes painful joint inflammation. Diuretics also may cause nausea, confusion, drowsiness, weakness (due to low blood pressure), and muscle or leg cramps. Report these and any other side effects to your doctor.

Digoxin

Digoxin is in a class of drugs known as cardiac glycosides. It helps a weakened heart contract more strongly by inhibiting an enzyme called adenosine triphosphatase (ATPase) in heart cells. More importantly, digoxin inhibits ATPase in the kidneys and the central nervous system, which decreases neurohormonal activation. For this reason, digoxin is classified as a neurohormonal modulating agent.

Digoxin improves symptoms, functional capacity, exercise tolerance, and quality of life in patients with heart failure. It also can reduce hospitalizations for worsening heart failure, particularly in people with an ejection fraction of less than 25 percent. However, digoxin does not improve survival.

Digoxin Side Effects. Digoxin is available as tablets (Lanoxin, Digitek), a pediatric elixir (Lanoxin Pediatric), liquid-filled capsules (Lanoxicaps), or a liquid used for injection (Lanoxin Injection).

Oral digoxin usually is taken once daily on a regular schedule, and a low dose—0.125 milligrams (mg)—is effective in most patients. Lower doses are used in the frail elderly and people with kidney dysfunction. Occasionally, higher doses may be used in people with arrhythmias. Doctors consider the patient's weight, kidney function, age, cardiac medications, and the presence of other diseases when choosing a dose. High doses can be toxic. To maintain a digoxin level less than 1.0 mg per milliliter (ml), regular monitoring is needed. When the dosage of digoxin is optimal, side effects are uncommon. At higher doses, side effects may include cardiac arrhythmias, gastrointestinal problems, such as nausea and vomiting, and neurologic problems, such as vision changes, headache, fatigue, and confusion. If you experience such side effects, contact your doctor immediately.

Certain drugs can decrease the effect of digoxin or increase its concentration to a potentially dangerous level. If you are taking antacids, kaolin-pectin (Kaopectate), Milk of Magnesia, or the anti-rheumatic drug sulfasalazine (Azulfidine), allow as much time as possible between taking these drugs and digoxin. When digoxin is taken with clarithromycin (Biaxin), erythromycin (Erythrocin), amiodarone (Cordarone, Pacerone), itraconazole (Onmel, Sporanox), cyclosporine (Neoral, Restasis), or verapamil (Calan), the digoxin dose must be reduced.

Like any drug, digoxin should be taken exactly as directed. Withdrawal from digoxin can result in a worsening of symptoms, so most people with heart failure must take the drug for as long as their symptoms persist.

Aldosterone Antagonists

Aldosterone is a hormone secreted by the adrenal glands. Its main function is to signal the kidneys to retain sodium and water. Spironolactone (Aldactone) and eplerenone (Inspra) are weak diuretics that also block the hormone aldosterone from interacting with its receptor.

Aldosterone antagonists are prescribed primarily to help patients eliminate excess water, but they have the ability to reverse left-ventricular remodeling and improve survival in people with heart failure.

The usual starting dose of spironolactone for severe heart failure symptoms is 12.5 to 25 mg per day. Patients with kidney dysfunction (creatinine levels above 2.5 mg per deciliter [dL], or high blood potassium levels (greater than 5.0 mg/dL) should not take the drug. Kidney function and potassium levels must be monitored regularly in all patients taking spironolactone.

Eplerenone is approved for the prevention of heart failure following a heart attack in patients with a history of heart failure or an ejection fraction of 40 percent or less. A major 2003 study demonstrated that eplerenone reduced deaths and hospitalizations in people who had experienced a recent heart attack and had evidence of heart failure or low ejection fraction.

Aldosterone Antagonist Side Effects. Aldosterone is a steroid hormone and a mineralocorticoid. Other steroid hormones regulate sugar metabolism (glucocorticoids) and sexual characteristics (estrogens and androgens) by interacting with their own receptors. Because steroid hormones share certain molecular characteristics, aldosterone also can

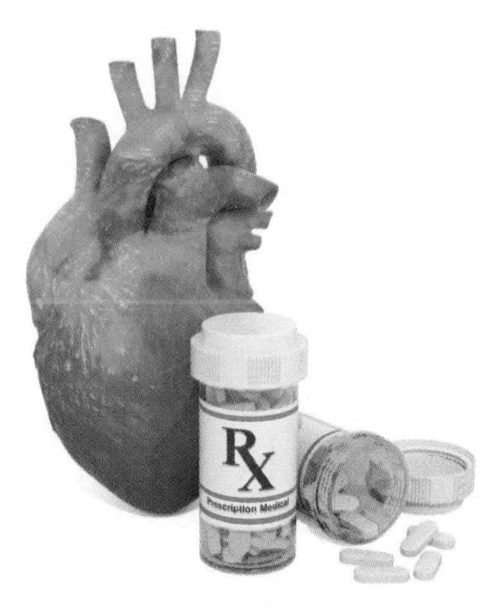

Early treatment of heart failure is known to slow its progression.

interact with receptors for glucocorticoids, estrogens, and androgens. This is why spironolactone can cause gynecomastia (breast enlargement in men). Because eplerenone blocks only the mineralocorticoid aldosterone receptor, it does not cause gynecomastia.

Patients with impaired kidney function should not take aldosterone antagonists due to the increased risk for elevated potassium levels.

Hydralazine Plus a Nitrate

Nitrates release nitric oxide, which dilates your arteries and veins. Hydralazine causes small arteries to dilate and independently lowers blood pressure. In addition, it appears to preserve nitrate's effectiveness, which can wane over time. Together, the two drugs improve hemodynamics (blood flow), lower blood pressure, and relieve symptoms. Studies confirm that the drug combination reverses remodeling and improves the heart's performance.

The combination of hydralazine plus a nitrate (Imdur, Isodil, Nitro-Patch) may be considered primary therapy for heart failure in African-American patients. It also is approved as an add-on therapy for any patient who continues to experience the symptoms of NYHA class III heart failure while taking ACE inhibitors, digoxin, beta-blockers, and spironolactone. The combination also may be useful in patients whose kidneys do not function well or who develop elevated potassium levels and cannot tolerate ACE inhibitors or ARBs.

Hydralazine Side Effects. Hydralazine may cause flushing, headaches, loss of appetite, nausea and vomiting, diarrhea, constipation, watery eyes, nasal congestion, and a rash. Report these side effects to your doctor if they persist.

More severe side effects include joint or muscle pain, tingling in the hands and feet, swollen ankles and feet, a rapid heartbeat, chest pain, and fever. If you experience these symptoms while you are taking hydralazine, you should call your doctor immediately.

Intravenous Vasodilators

Conventional intravenous vasodilators include nesiritide (Natrecor), nitroglycerin (Nitrostat), and nitroprusside (Nitropress). These medications are used to dilate arteries and veins in critically ill heart failure patients.

Currently, nesiritide is used at the physician's discretion. Intravenous nitroglycerin is generally started in the hospital emergency department and continued in the intensive care unit. An oral form of the drug may be given for use after discharge. Nitroprusside is used in patients with severe heart failure to improve symptoms, relieve congestion, lower blood pressure, and increase cardiac output. When this powerful arterial and venous dilator is used, patients must be carefully monitored to avoid hypotension (low blood pressure). Nitroprusside is rarely used outside the intensive care unit.

Intravenous Vasodilator Side Effects. Possible side effects include flushing, rash, itching, hives, nausea and vomiting, blurred vision, and difficulty breathing or swallowing. Report these symptoms to your doctor immediately.

Intravenous Inotropes

Intravenous inotropes include dobutamine and milrinone. They are used in critically ill heart failure patients with shock, low blood pressure, or low cardiac output. Intravenous inotropes also are given to patients awaiting heart transplantation, and are used as continuous palliative therapy to improve quality of life for end-stage heart failure patients who wish to remain at home.

Intravenous inotropes are not recommended for the routine treatment

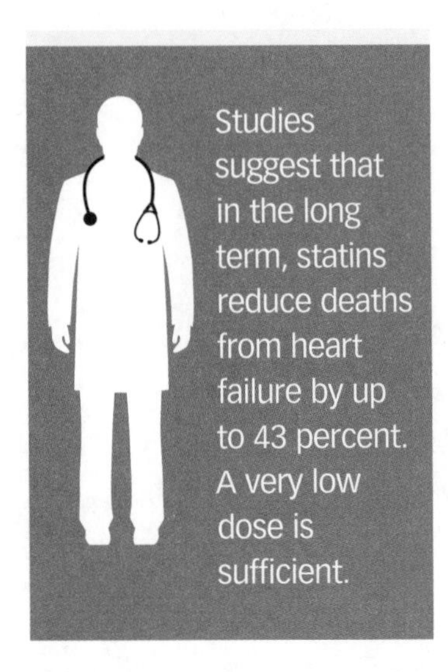

of acute decompensated heart failure, due to lack of long-term benefit and increased risk of complications such as low blood pressure, abnormal heart rhythms, and death. Intermittent infusions of these agents also are discouraged, since no clinical trials have demonstrated benefit.

Intravenous Inotrope Side Effects. These may include headaches and nausea. More serious side effects, such as a slow or rapid heartbeat, chest pain, and difficulty breathing, should be reported to your doctor immediately.

Atrial Fibrillation

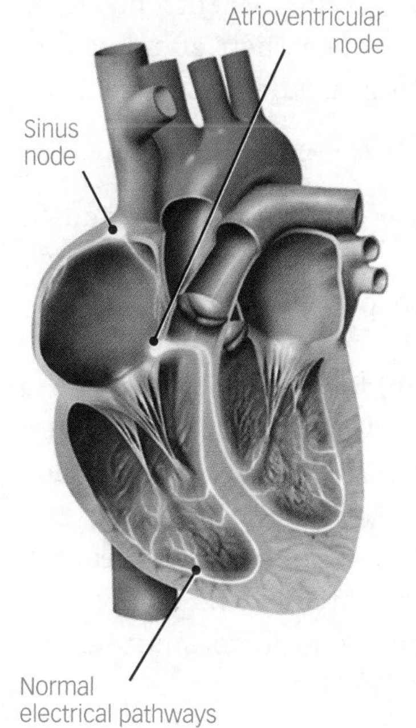

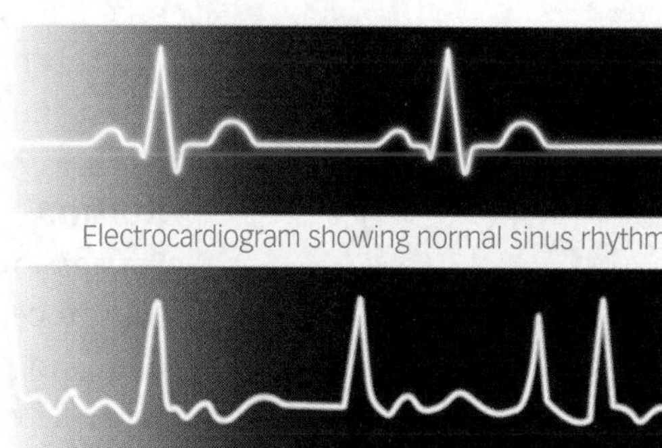

Each contraction of the heart muscle is controlled by an electrical signal that originates in a group of cells called the sinus node and travels through the upper chambers of the heart (atria) to the lower chambers of the heart (ventricles) via the atrioventricular node. In atrial fibrillation, the electrical signal becomes chaotic. This causes the upper atria to beat in a rapid, irregular manner that prevents the heart from pumping properly.

Other Drugs Used in Heart Failure

A range of other drugs may be used in people with heart failure who have abnormal heart rhythms, low levels of certain electrolytes, and/or high cholesterol levels.

Anti-Arrhythmia Medications

People with heart failure can develop one of two heart rhythm abnormalities: supraventricular arrhythmia or ventricular arrhythmia. The most common supraventricular arrhythmia is atrial fibrillation (A-fib), which occurs in up to 30 percent of people with heart failure. A-fib causes the atrial muscle cells to contract in a rapid, disorganized manner. This prevents the heart from filling properly, and cardiac output can drop by as much as 20 percent from the loss of normal rhythm. A-fib also increases the risk of a blood clot (thrombus), which can cause a stroke, peripheral embolism, or pulmonary embolism.

A-fib may resolve spontaneously, but if it continues to occur, an anti-arrhythmia drug may be given. However, because many anti-arrhythmia drugs can be dangerous for people with heart failure, a procedure called ablation may be used instead. In studies comparing medications to ablation, ablation was far more successful at helping patients remain alive, active, arrhythmia-free, and out of the hospital.

Ventricular arrhythmias, such as ventricular fibrillation and ventricular tachycardia are known to increase the risk of sudden death. Unfortunately, efforts to suppress these arrhythmias with drug therapy have been disappointing. Surgically implanted defibrillators that monitor heart rhythm often are needed. These do a better job than anti-arrhythmia medications at preventing sudden death in people with ventricular arrhythmias.

Potassium and Magnesium Supplements

One risk of diuretic therapy is low potassium and/or magnesium levels, which increase the likelihood of dying from an arrhythmia. Fortunately, these conditions are easily corrected with potassium or magnesium supplements. Low potassium is less likely to occur in people taking ACE inhibitors and spironolactone or eplerenone. In fact, high

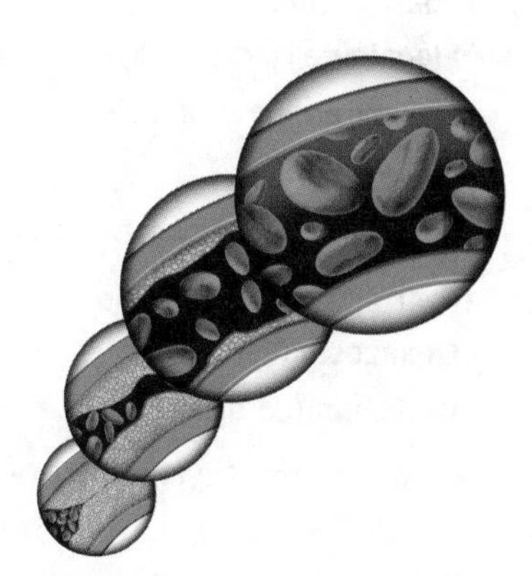

Statins are effective at helping prevent the buildup of fatty plaque in the arteries.

levels of potassium can occur with aldosterone blockers—as such, people who take potassium supplements may need to stop or reduce their supplements when starting an aldosterone blocker.

Statins

Statins lower cholesterol levels and, in the process, reduce heart attacks and death in people with elevated cholesterol. They also have other beneficial effects, including the ability to reduce inflammatory factors and cytokines, improve endothelial function, and stabilize plaque. However, there is little data that statins reduce the risk of death in heart failure patients who do not have elevated cholesterol, coronary artery disease, or diabetes.

In terms of preventing heart failure, the longer statins are taken, the greater the benefit: In studies, the impact of statins on heart failure appeared after five years of use. After 15 years, the drugs reduced deaths from heart failure by a whopping 43 percent. A very low dose appears to be sufficient. Higher doses do not offer better protection, but do increase the risk of side effects. Studies also have found that statins had a more powerful effect than ACE inhibitors and beta-blockers on survival rates in patients with diastolic heart failure. Although ACE inhibitors and beta-blockers are traditionally used in heart failure, one- and three-year mortality rates were lower among people who were taking statins, regardless of their age, total cholesterol level, or the presence of coronary artery disease, diabetes, or hypertension. Nevertheless, the use of statins in heart failure appears to be most beneficial in the early stages of the disease—studies have failed to show a benefit by adding statins in later stages.

Emerging Therapies

There is an urgent need to discover more effective medications to remove salt and water from the body, and relax arteries. The need is particularly acute for people who have decompensated

Drugs to Avoid if You Have Heart Failure

These drugs should not be used, or should be used with caution, by patients with heart failure:

Diabetes Medications

- Thiazolidinediones, particularly **pioglitazone** (Actos)
- Dipeptidyl peptidase-4 inhibitors

Antiarrhythmics

- **Flecainide** (Tambocor)
- **Disopyramide** (Norpace)
- **Sotalol** (Betapace)
- **Dronedarone** (Multaq)

Cancer Drugs

- Many—physicians weigh the benefits against the risks

Hypertension Medications

- **Doxazosin** (Cardura)
- **Diltiazem** (Cardizem)
- **Verapamil** (Calan)
- **Moxonidine** (Physiotens)

Neurologic and Psychiatric Drugs

- Stimulants
- Appetite suppressants
- **Pergolide** (Permax, Prascend)
- **Pramipexole** (Mirapex)

Nonsteroidal Anti-Inflammatory Drugs (NSAIDs)

- **Ibuprofen** (Advil, Motrin)
- **Diclofenac** (Cataflam, Voltaren)
- **Celecoxib** (Celebrex)
- **Sulindac** (Clinoril)
- **Indomethacin** (Indocin)
- **Naproxen** (Aleve, Naprosyn)

Decongestants

- **Pseudoephedrine** (Sudafed)

Pulmonary Drugs

- **Albuterol** (ProAir HFA, Proventil HFA)
- **Bosentan** (Tracleer)
- **Epoprostenol** (Veletri, Flolan)

Rheumatology Drugs

- TNF-a inhibitors, such as **adalimumab** (Humira), (etanercept (Enbrel), and **infliximab** (Remicade) heart failure, because no drug has been shown to deliver long-term positive results. Cleveland Clinic physicians and other researchers around the world are conducting clinical trials of many new agents developed to relieve symptoms and prevent complications. One drug with potential is sildenafil (Viagra, Revatio). Sildenafil offers a number of benefits in heart failure with pulmonary hypertension. Specifically, it allows patients to breathe better, and in one study, it also reduced hospitalizations for heart failure. The drug also appears to limit heart remodeling, in effect slowing the deterioration process that is the hallmark of heart failure.

Vasopressin antagonists ("aquaretics") have the potential to remove fluid and decrease congestion without adversely affecting blood pressure, heart rate, electrolyte levels, or kidney function. In other words, they do the work of diuretics without upsetting body chemistry. Although the vasopressin antagonist tolvaptan (Samsca) failed to improve survival in clinical trials, the drug was approved for short-term treatment of hyponatremia (low sodium levels). Use of this drug is limited, however, by its high cost and its potential to cause serious liver damage.

Sodium-glucose cotransporter 2 (SGLT2) inhibitors are used to treat type 2 diabetes, and include empagliflozin (Jardiance), canagliflozin (Invokana), dapagliflozin (Farxiga), and ertugliflozin (Steglatro). In clinical trials leading to the FDA approval of these drugs for their effect on blood glucose levels, three (all but ertugliflozin) were discovered to have cardiovascular benefits. In particular, dapagliflozin was shown to benefit heart failure (see "Diabetes Drug Improves Heart Failure Outcomes").

Drugs to Avoid

The following drugs are detrimental to people with heart failure and should be stopped or used with great caution:

NSAIDs

This class of common painkillers, available over the counter and by prescription, includes ibuprofen (Advil, Motrin), naproxen (Aleve, Naprosyn), and celecoxib (Celebrex). If it is necessary for you to take NSAIDs, your cardiologist will want to monitor you closely.

Diabetes Medications

Diabetes medications in the thiazolidinedione class, such as pioglitazone (Actos), may increase edema (tissue swelling) in people with heart failure. Some physicians have not found the risk to be excessive, and feel that the advantages of this drug may outweigh its risks. If you have heart failure and are taking this medication, your doctor may not stop the drug, but may instead monitor you closely.

The risk of heart failure may increase with saxagliptin (Onglyza), alogliptin (Nesina), saxagliptin plus extended-release metformin (Kombiglyze XR), alogliptin plus metformin (Kazano), and alogliptin plus pioglitazone (Oseni). The risk is particularly high in people who have existing cardiovascular or kidney disease.

Saxagliptin and alogliptin are dipeptidyl-peptidase 4 (DPP-4) inhibitors. A large trial conducted with sitagliptin (Januvia), a third member of the same class of drugs, found no increased risk for heart failure in people with type 2 diabetes. Nevertheless, the AHA lists both sitagliptin and saxagliptin, but not alogliptin, in its list of drugs that may cause or exacerbate heart failure.

NEW FINDING

Diabetes Drug Improves Heart Failure Outcomes

There are many different drugs for lowering blood glucose levels in diabetes, but none are as effective on heart health as the new class of drugs called sodium-glucose cotransporter 2 (SGLT2) inhibitors. At this time, four are available in the United States, and several more are in clinical trials.

Empagliflozin (Jardiance) was the first SGL2 inhibitor to show a reduced risk of cardiovascular death in patients with diabetes and known cardiovascular disease. Similarly, canagliflozin (Invokana) reduced the risk of stroke, heart attack, and cardiovascular death in the same group of patients.

But it's dapagliflozin (Farxiga) that appears to benefit heart failure. In a clinical trial known as Dapagliflozin Effect on Cardiovascular Events (DECLARE-TIMI-58), the drug reduced the composite end point of heart-failure hospitalization and cardiovascular death by 38 percent in people with heart failure with reduced ejection fraction (HFrEF) and an ejection fraction less than 45 percent. Among all HFrEF patients, all-cause mortality dropped 41 percent.

Circulation, May 28, 2019

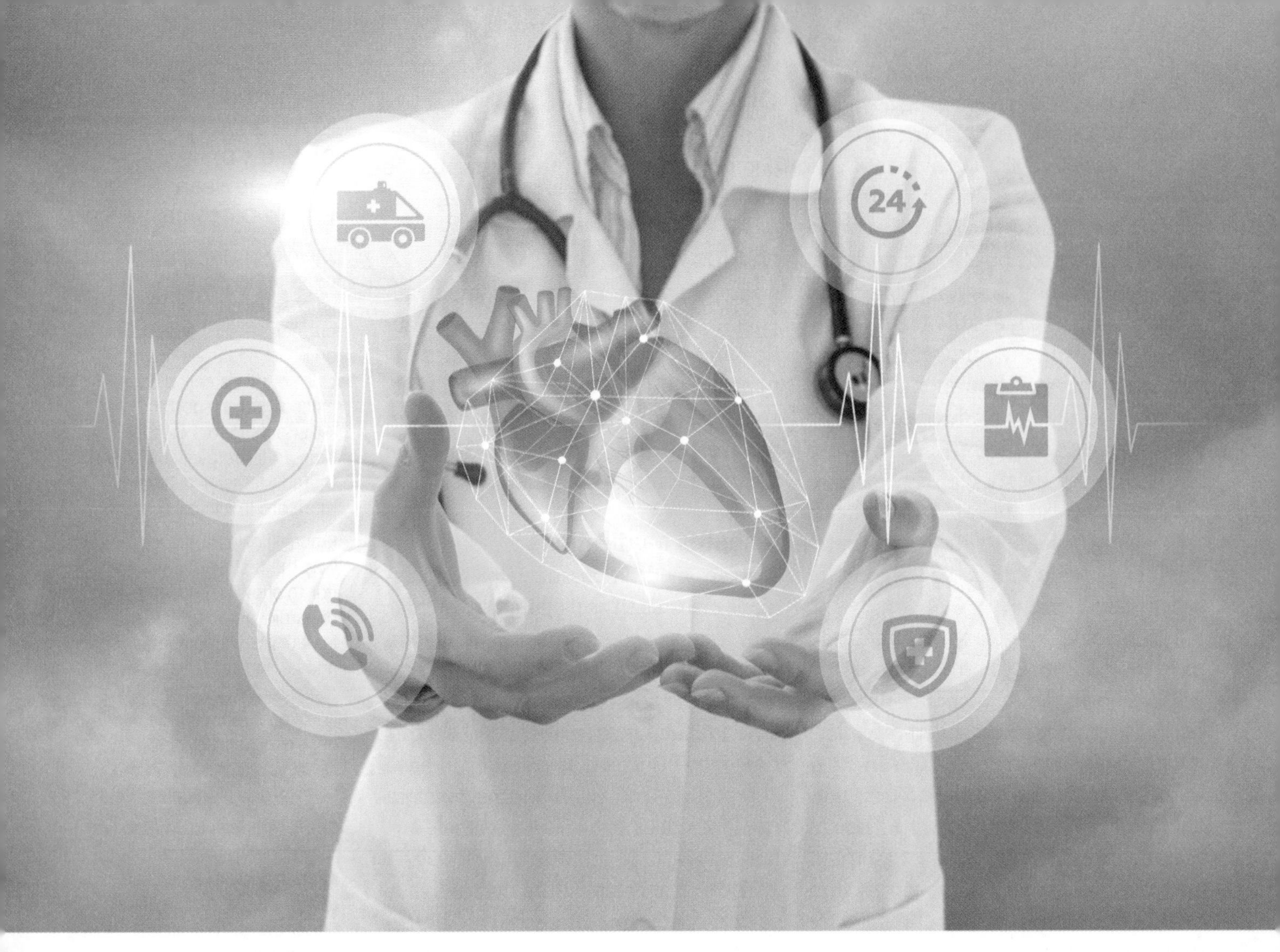

© Nataliia Mysik | Dreamstime

Some people with heart failure require advanced treatments to maintain their quality of life.

8 Advanced Treatments for Heart Failure

When fatty plaques severely narrow the coronary arteries, coronary artery bypass surgery or angioplasty with stenting can improve blood flow to heart tissue and improve heart function. Floppy, leaky valves and stiff, calcified valves can be repaired or replaced. Underlying congenital defects or aneurysms can be repaired. These treatments often improve heart failure.

Sometimes, however, these interventions are not enough, and additional help is needed. Advanced options for treating heart failure generally fall into five categories: ultrafiltration, electronic device therapy, mechanical circulatory support, surgical procedures, and heart transplantation. Innovative devices are opening up a new world of possibilities.

Ultrafiltration

Ultrafiltration (also known as aquapheresis) is a method of extracting water from the body in a process similar to dialysis. It sometimes is used in patients admitted to the hospital with fluid overload, edema, and ascites (buildup of fluid in the abdomen) from acute decompensated heart failure.

Ultrafiltration removes more sodium and water than intravenous diuretics without causing kidney dysfunction or elevated potassium levels. The fact that ultrafiltration is more expensive than loop diuretic infusions and requires large intravenous catheters prevents its widespread use. Cleveland Clinic cardiologists use ultrafiltration when patients need to unload very large amounts of fluid caused by acute decompensated heart failure.

Electronic Device Therapy

Used alongside drugs, pacemakers and cardioverter defibrillators have extended and improved the lives of many people with heart failure.

Cardiac Resynchronization Therapy

The heart is most efficient when its beat is synchronized—that is, the outside wall (free wall) of the left ventricle and the wall that divides the left and right ventricles (septum) squeeze toward each other to eject blood. In heart failure, and particularly in dilated cardiomyopathy, the electrical signals that stimulate the heart to contract fail to follow the right path, because scar tissue from a heart attack blocks the path or the ventricle walls have stretched out. In about 30 percent of patients with this condition, the free wall and septum of the left ventricle move out of synch, making ejection more difficult. This is called dyssynchrony, and it causes the ejection fraction to drop and heart failure to worsen.

Cardiac resynchronization therapy (CRT) is a method of making the ventricles contract properly with a pacemaker. Pacemakers prevent a heart from beating too slowly. They are set at a minimum number of beats per minute, and if the heart rate drops below this level, the pacemaker stimulates the heart to beat faster.

A biventricular pacemaker may be used in people with heart failure. The device usually is implanted below the collarbone. Three electrodes are threaded into the heart through a vein and positioned in the right atrium, right ventricle, and left cardiac vein. The electrodes are programmed to stimulate both sides of the heart to contract at the same time. The frequency and timing are adjusted to produce a more efficient heartbeat. The procedure improves heart function, resulting in less need for diuretics. CRT also improves heart failure symptoms and quality of life and reduces complications and risk of sudden death. It also may improve left ventricular function, and it reverses remodeling in some individuals.

CRT is an accepted treatment for people with moderate-to-severe heart failure who fall into New York Heart Association (NYHA) classes III and IV. In these patients, CRT increases the efficiency of the heart, reduces symptoms and improves survival and quality of life.

In people with mild heart failure and left bundle branch block (LBBB, a problem with the heart's electrical system), CRT with a defibrillator (CRT-D) can reduce the likelihood of dying or suffering a nonfatal heart attack.

Cardiac Resynchronization Therapy

In cardiac resynchronization therapy, cardiologists use a special pacemaker to pace both ventricles. The pacemaker is usually implanted in the left front chest below the collarbone and is connected to electrodes that are threaded into the heart through a vein. The electrodes are programmed to stimulate both sides of the heart simultaneously, so that they contract in synchrony.

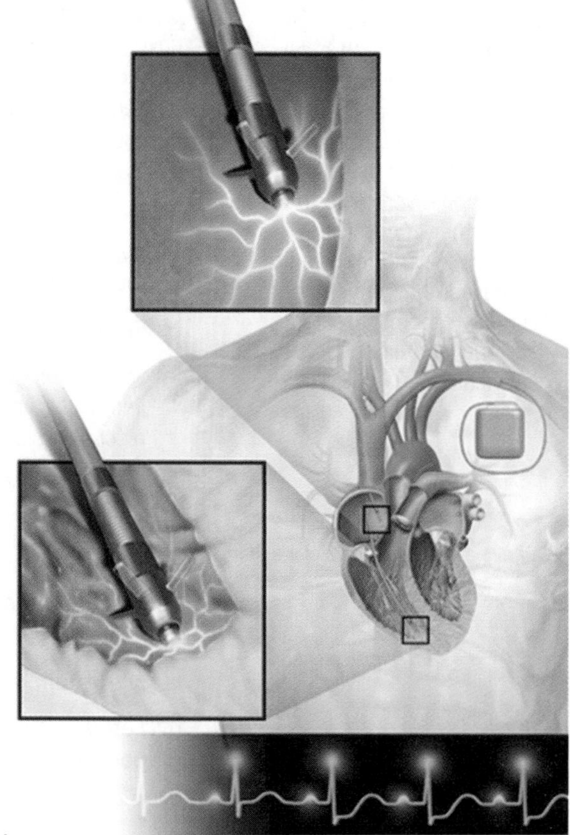

NEW FINDING

New Therapy Optimizes Cardiac Output

In March 2019, the U.S. Food and Drug Administration (FDA) approved a pacemaker-type device for patients with moderate-to-severe heart failure who don't qualify for cardiac resynchronization therapy. Such patients have narrow QRS intervals on electrocardiography and a left ventricular ejection fraction of 25 to 45 percent.

The new device, called the Optimizer Smart System, delivers electrical pulses to specific sites in the heart during the heartbeat. This action does not affect heart rhythm like a standard pacemaker does. Instead, it changes the chemistry inside heart cells. With long-term use, this process—called cardiac contractility modulation—improves the heart's ability to contract.

In clinical trials leading to the Optimizer's designation by the FDA as a Breakthrough Device (which expedited its review process), people who received the Optimizer in addition to heart-failure medications were able to walk farther in physical fitness tests, and reported a decrease in how much heart-failure symptoms affected their quality of life and daily activities.

FDA Device Approval, March 21, 2019

Cardiac Contractility Modulation

About 30 percent of people with heart failure do not respond to biventricular pacing, including those with moderate-to-severe heart failure and a narrow QRS interval (<150 milliseconds—for more on this, see Chapter 5). For these patients, cardiac contractility modulation with the Optimizer Smart System is a new option (see "New Therapy Optimizes Cardiac Output").

Implantable Cardioverter Defibrillators

About half of all heart failure patients die suddenly from cardiac arrest. That's why some heart failure patients receive an implantable cardioverter defibrillator, or ICD. This device monitors the heart's rhythm with leads implanted in the right atrium and right ventricle. When it detects the potentially deadly heart rhythm called ventricular fibrillation, it either paces the heart or delivers a shock that restores the heart's normal rhythm.

ICDs are highly effective, but the shocks can be painful. If the heart must be shocked often, an alternative (such as medication or ablation) is generally advised. A less painful method of shocking the heart into rhythm involves employing five to 10 fast pacemaker pulses called a burst. In appropriately selected patients, this technique, called anti-tachycardia pacing, causes the heart rate to return to normal.

ICDs showed their superiority over standard medical therapy with amiodarone (Cordarone, Pacerone) in the landmark Sudden Cardiac Death in Heart Failure Trial (SCD-HeFT). In this trial, the ICDs were programmed to shock the heart when necessary but not to pace it. The goal was to evaluate which treatment would improve

Implantable Cardioverter Defibrillator Guidelines

Data from clinical trials, such as the Sudden Cardiac Death in Heart Failure Trial (SCD-HeFT), have enabled organizations to write guidelines for who might benefit from receiving an implantable cardioverter defibrillator (ICD). There are some differences among guidelines written by the American College of Cardiology/American Heart Association (ACC/AHA), the European Society of Cardiology, and the Canadian Cardiovascular Society. ACC/AHA guidelines are below.

ICD therapy is recommended for patients who have:

- ☑ Spontaneous sustained ventricular tachycardia
- ☑ Survived cardiac arrest
- ☑ Inducible ventricular tachycardia/ventricular fibrillation in the electrophysiology laboratory
- ☑ A familial or inherited condition with a high risk of life-threatening ventricular tachyarrhythmia
- ☑ Post-myocardial infarction (MI), left ventricular dysfunction

The Centers for Medicare & Medicaid Services guidelines for ICD implantation require that the following conditions be met to ensure reimbursement:

Ischemic Cardiomyopathy

- ☑ **Waiting period:** 40 days from MI, 90 days from bypass or angioplasty
- ☑ **NYHA functional class:** I to IV*
- ☑ **Left ventricular ejection fraction:** ≤35 percent

Dilated Cardiomyopathy

- ☑ **Waiting period:** Nine months from diagnosis (may differ from symptom onset)
- ☑ **NYHA functional class:** II to IV**

*NYHA class IV patients must be eligible for cardiac resynchronization therapy.
**NYHA class I patients with dilated cardiomyopathy do not qualify for ICD.

the prognosis by reducing deaths due to heart arrhythmias.

The study participants were evaluated for more than two years. Of the 829 with an ICD, 259 received shocks from the device, and 68 percent of these were for life-threatening ventricular tachycardia or ventricular fibrillation. ICDs were found to reduce the risk of sudden death by 23 percent, whereas amiodarone offered no survival benefit. As a result of this trial, the standard of care changed in favor of ICD therapy, despite a 5 percent rate of device-related complications.

The SCD-HeFT trial held some surprises. Patients with milder (NYHA class II) disease benefited greatly from the ICD, but the device failed to help sicker patients (NYHA class III). ICDs also tended to work better in patients who had ejection fractions of 30 percent or less, were able to walk six minutes on a treadmill, were under age 65, did not have diabetes, and were taking beta-blockers. Since exercise does not trigger shocks, patients with ICDs are able to exercise, which improves their overall health and quality of life.

Implantable Cardioverter Defibrillator

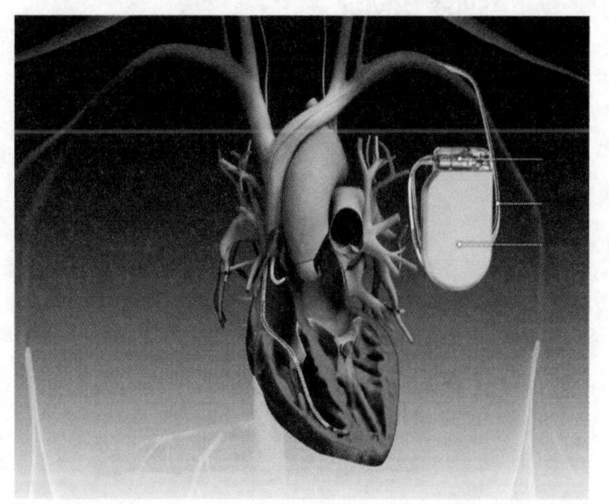

An implantable cardioverter defibrillator incorporates a pulse generator that is placed under the skin of the chest, and electrodes that are positioned in the right atrium and right ventricle. When needed, the device delivers a mild electric shock to pace the heart or restore normal rhythm.

Mechanical Circulatory Support

Physicians and researchers in Cleveland Clinic's Kaufman Center for Heart Failure have leadership roles in the Interagency Registry for Mechanically Assisted Circulatory Support (INTERMACS). INTERMACS is a national registry of patients with advanced heart failure whose treatment includes a mechanical circulatory support device that has been approved by the U.S. Food and Drug Administration (FDA).

INTERMACS was created through a joint effort of the National Heart, Lung, and Blood Institute, the Centers for Medicare & Medicaid Services, the FDA, clinicians, scientists, and industry representatives in conjunction with the University of Alabama at Birmingham and United Network for Organ Sharing (UNOS). All patients who receive an advanced device are registered in the database. The information gathered will help heart failure experts determine which patients are most likely to benefit from which devices and identify the factors determining whether an outcome will be good or poor, as well as develop best-practice guidelines that minimize complications. The information also is used to guide the development of new devices.

Ventricular Assist Devices

When maximum medical therapy no longer controls heart failure symptoms, ventricular assist devices (VADs) become an option. Cleveland Clinic has one of the oldest and most active VAD programs in the country. It is one of the few programs offering a variety of FDA-approved left (systolic) heart failure VADs (LVADs). This enables Cleveland Clinic surgeons to choose the device that best suits each patient's needs.

VADs were pioneered in the 1970s, but they were not widely used until the 1990s as a way to keep patients alive during their wait for a heart transplant ("bridge to transplant"). They still are

Experience Counts with Ventricular Assist Devices

The success of a ventricular assist device (VAD) depends to a large degree on the experience and expertise of the implantation team. Research suggests that outcomes are better in approved VAD centers that implant more than four VADs per year. One reason for the better outcomes appears to be that these centers are better at managing extremely ill heart failure patients. Cleveland Clinic routinely implants between 80 and 100 VADs every year.

The HeartMate 3™ Ventricular Assist Device

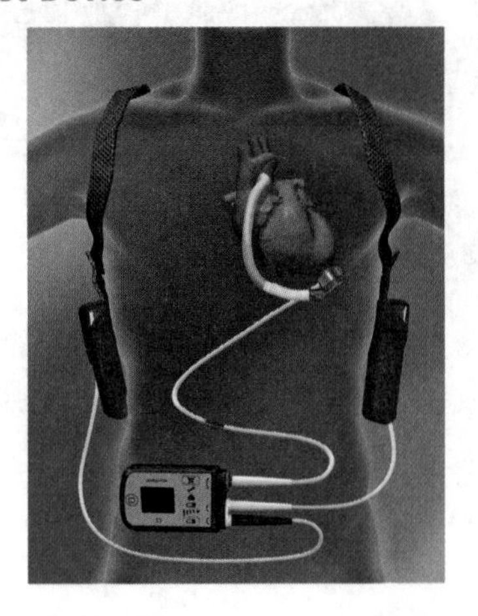

© Thoratec Corp.

The newest ventricular assist devices (VADs), like the HeartMate 3, keep patients with advanced heart failure out of the hospital and allow them to go about their daily lives. The HeartMate 3, like the HeartWare VAD, is approved by the U.S. Food and Drug Administration both as a bridge to transplant and as a permanent heart.

used for this purpose. Today they also are used as a permanent alternative in people who are not eligible for heart transplantation ("destination therapy").

A VAD supports the heart in pumping oxygenated blood throughout the body. A battery power pack enables a VAD wearer to be out and about for several hours. This allows weak patients with advanced heart failure to become more active and improve their health and fitness. Those waiting for a heart transplant are stronger and better able to withstand the stress of surgery when a donor heart becomes available.

One-tenth to one-third of patients on a VAD and optimal medical therapy may recover well enough to have the device removed, even if they had been waiting for a heart transplant or expecting to retain their VAD for life. This exciting development has earned VADs a third designation: that of "bridge to recovery." No matter the intention, however, VADs help patients feel better, have more energy, and enjoy a better quality of life.

An Evolving Technology. First-generation VADs were designed to pulse like a heart. They were powered by a cable connected to a power source in a battery pack worn at the waist or carried in a shoulder bag. These early VADs were prone to infection and blood clots that caused strokes, but over time, more biocompatible materials and innovative designs have overcome many complications. Second-generation VADs are totally implantable, continuous-flow ("axial-flow") pumps. They push blood in one direction, like water through a hose. The combination of a biocompatible design and new materials reduces the risk of blood clots, infections, and strokes, compared with older VADs.

The HeartMate II has been one of the most successful of these VADs—since 2008, its one-year survival rate has remained at 85 percent. For several years the HeartMate II was used both as a bridge to transplant and destination (final) therapy. It has since been replaced by the HeartMate 3, a miniaturized VAD with a single moving part that propels blood with a rotating turbine. Suspended by magnets, the turbine creates no friction. In the MOMENTUM 3 study, no difference in the rate of death or disabling stroke were seen between the HeartMate

The HeartWare® Ventricular Assist Device

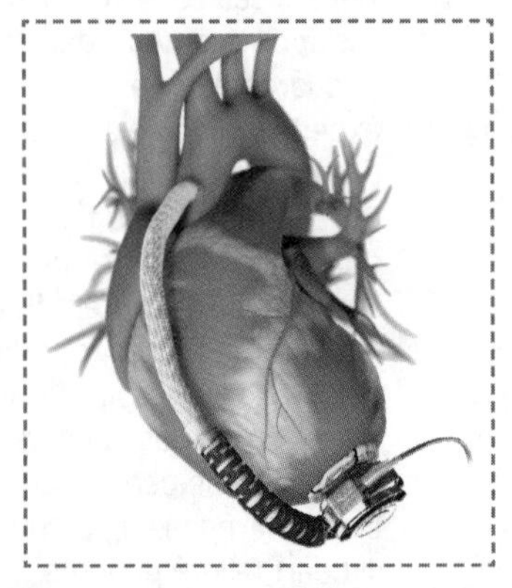

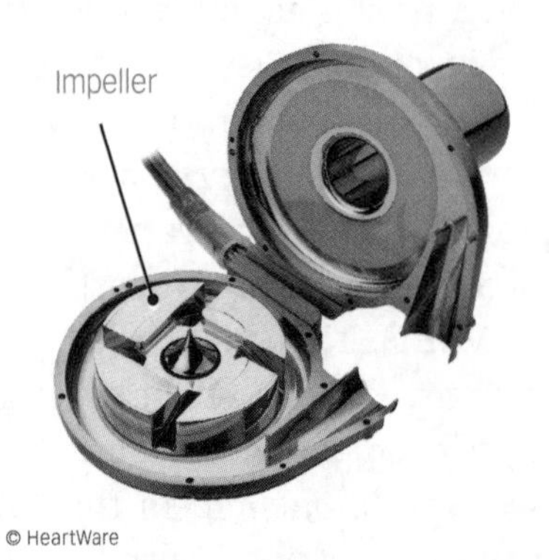

© HeartWare

Tiny third-generation ventricular assist devices, like the HeartWare model seen here, have a single moving part (called an impeller) that propels blood with a rotating turbine. The impeller is suspended by magnets, does not create friction, and has no parts to wear out.

II and HeartMate 3 at six months. At the two-year mark, 80 percent of patients with the HeartMate 3 survived stroke-free, compared with 60 percent of HeartMate II patients.

The HeartMate 3 and the HeartWare (another third-generation VAD) are highly biocompatible and resistant to wear and corrosion. These factors make them ideal for permanent use, especially with extended-life batteries that may be recharged using household current. As such, both VADs are approved by the FDA as destination therapy.

For people with HFrEF or HFpEF requiring temporary support, Cleveland Clinic also uses a unique device known as the Impella. A long tube, the Impella is inserted by catheter through the groin, into the heart, and across the aortic valve, where it rests in the left ventricle. As the heart pumps, a tiny turbine, which is the size of a ballpoint-pen spring and located inside the Impella, helps pull blood out of the ventricle into the atrium, where it is pumped into circulation.

Cleveland Clinic also uses the TandemHeart VAD to provide short-term support for the heart's pumping chamber in selected patients following heart surgery, during high-risk interventional procedures, and during electrophysiology procedures in which the left ventricle is being mapped.

Intra-Aortic Balloon Pump (IABP)

This mechanical assist device is inserted into the aorta through an artery in the groin. A balloon is located at the end of a catheter, and the opposite end is connected to a computer console. The IABP is programmed to inflate and deflate in sync with the patient's heartbeat. When the heart contracts, the balloon collapses, easing ejection. When the heart relaxes, the balloon inflates, causing blood flow in the aortic arch to reverse and blood flow to the coronary arteries to improve. Balloon pumps are used as temporary circulatory support in people with acute decompensated heart failure and cardiogenic shock (see "IABPs Improve Blood Flow").

Total Artificial Heart

Syncardia's Temporary Total Artificial Heart (TAH) has been used since 1993 as a bridge to transplant and has been

NEW FINDING

IABPs Improve Blood Flow

The intra-aortic balloon pump (IABP) is not a new device, but researchers are finding new uses for it. In a study of 32 adults who developed decompensated heart failure without suffering a heart attack, the IABP was better than intravenous inotropes (enoximone or dobutamine) at improving oxygen flow into the bloodstream and throughout the body. The device is similar in concept to Impella, but is less expensive and easier to implant.

Eurointervention, May 23, 2019

The Impella®

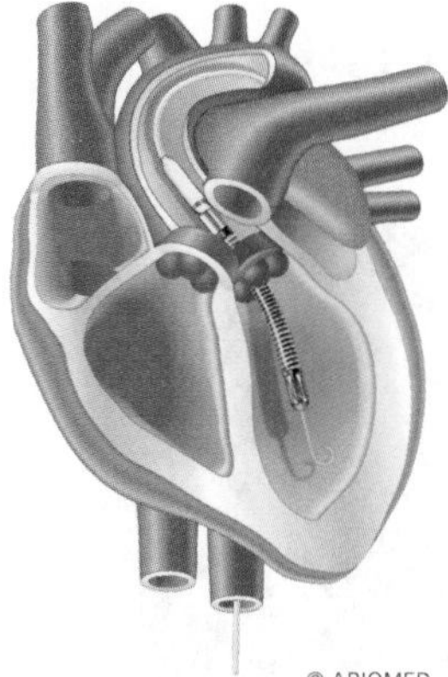

© ABIOMED

The temporary Impella device is inserted by catheter through the groin, into the heart and across the aortic valve, where it rests in the left ventricle. As the heart pumps, a tiny turbine, which is the size of a ballpoint pen spring and located inside the Impella, helps pull blood out of the ventricle into the aorta.

Intra-Aortic Balloon Pump

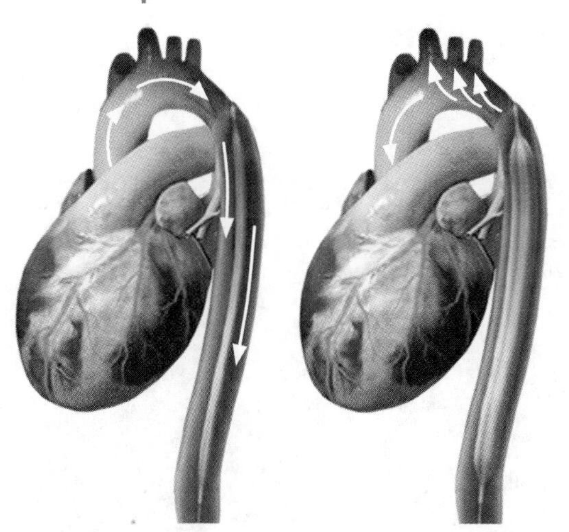

© Datascope Corp.

Intra-aortic balloon pumps work on a simple principle: When the heart contracts, the balloon collapses, easing ejection (left). When the heart relaxes, the balloon inflates, causing reversal of blood flow in the aortic arch and improving blood flow to the coronary arteries (right).

MitraClip™ Transcatheter Mitral Valve Repair System

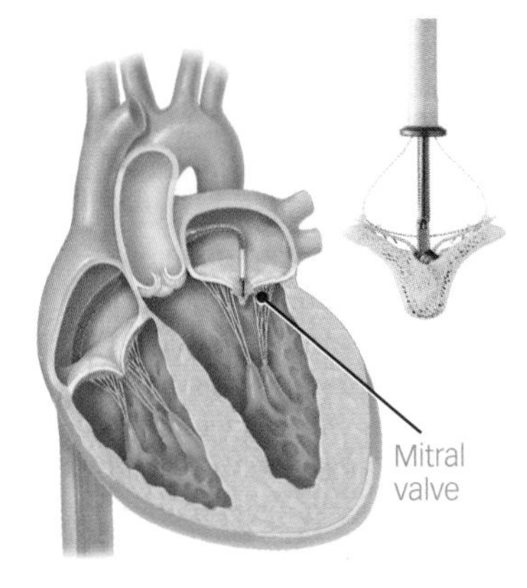

This tiny device is used to tighten the mitral valve and prevent mitral regurgitation.

implanted in more patients than any other total artificial heart. In 2004, the FDA approved the TAH for temporary use in eligible patients at risk of imminent death. The TAH completely replaces a failing heart and is designed to restore normal blood pressure and cardiac output. This improves circulation, which enables other organs that were jeopardized due to inadequate blood supply to recover. The result is that patients are better able to withstand and recover from a heart transplant.

Surgical Procedures

Surgery may be an option for patients with mitral valve disease or advanced coronary artery disease who are not helped by medications or angioplasty.

Mitral Valve Repair

In a remodeled heart, an enlarging left ventricle can strain the muscles and cords connected to the mitral valve. This distorts the valve's leaflets and prevents them from closing tightly between beats. The result is that blood flows backwards into the left atrium, further overloading the heart. The condition, called mitral regurgitation, is associated with increased risk of hospitalization, poor quality of life, and death from heart failure.

Previously, the benefits of repairing or replacing a mitral valve damaged by heart failure did not outweigh the risks. Then in 2018, researchers showed that repairing the valve in a minimally invasive procedure could be effective and safer. In this procedure, a tiny device called a MitraClip was introduced into the heart through a catheter and clipped onto the underside of the mitral valve to tighten it. In a landmark study, people who received the MitraClip had fewer hospitalizations (160 versus 183) and deaths (29.1 percent versus 46.1 percent) in 24 months than those who were treated medically. Few MitraClip patients experienced any device-related complication. Their degree of mitral regurgitation, left ventricular remodeling, and quality of life improved, along with their ability to walk further without becoming breathless.

Coronary Artery Bypass Grafting

Coronary artery disease (CAD) plays a significant role in HFrEF (see "Causes of Heart Failure," Chapter 2). Even when it is not the primary cause, CAD can

Coronary Artery Bypass Grafting

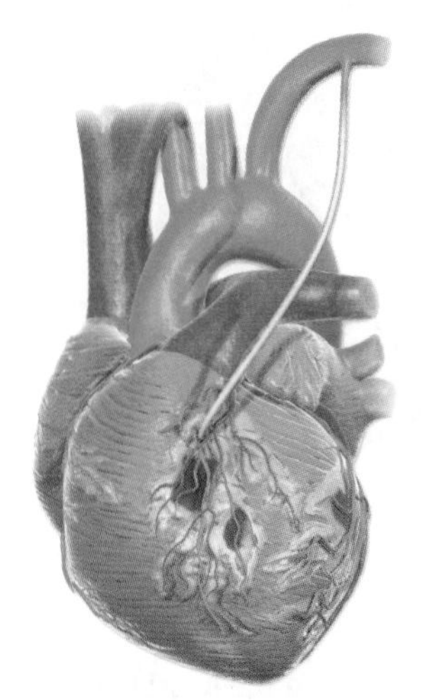

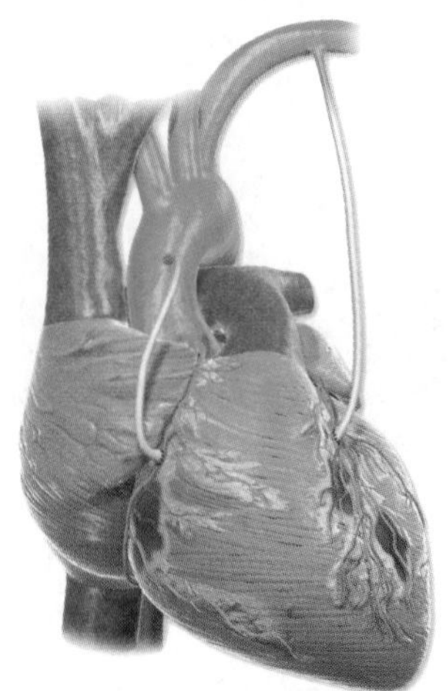

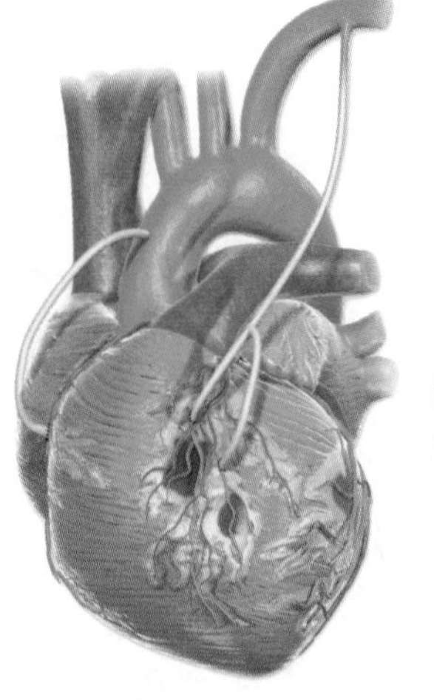

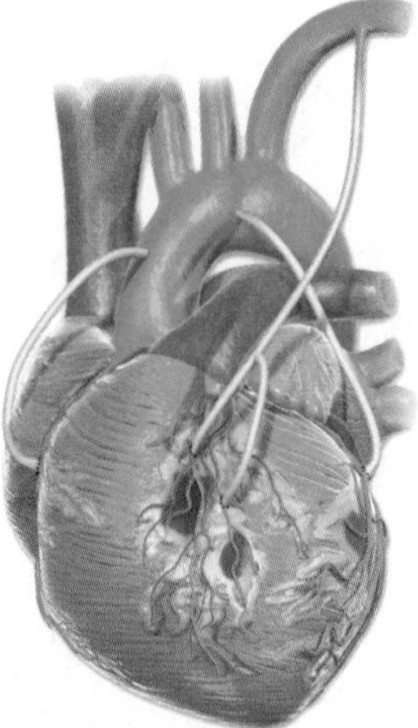

In coronary artery bypass grafting (CABG), blocked arteries are bypassed by the addition of grafted blood vessels from elsewhere in the body. It's common for three or four coronary arteries to be bypassed during CABG surgery.

prevent the heart from pumping optimally. When CAD causes significant loss of blood flow to the heart muscle (ischemia), coronary artery bypass grafting (CABG) often is used to improve blood flow and relieve symptoms.

The Surgical Treatment for Ischemic Heart Failure (STICH) trial, reported in 2011, showed that benefits of CABG in these patients outweighed the risks. In this study, patients ages 53 to 68 were treated with medications alone or with medications plus CABG. CABG increased the risk of death within two years. After two years, however, deaths in patients on medical therapy alone grew. During the five-year study, fewer CABG patients died from cardiovascular causes or required hospitalization for heart-related causes than those on medications alone.

Heart Transplantation

Heart transplantation remains the gold-standard treatment for end-stage heart failure because it has proven to be the most effective treatment. More than half of all patients who are transplanted survive more than 12 years. Unfortunately, the efficacy of this treatment is limited by an insufficient supply of donor hearts. An estimated 20,000 to 70,000 people per year in the United States could benefit from a heart transplant, yet in 2018 only 3,408 patients received one. Of these, 54 heart transplants were done at Cleveland Clinic.

The good news is that recent advances in medical and VAD therapy mean that transplantation is no longer the sole option in end-stage heart failure.

Who Is Suitable? Due to the organ shortage, heart transplantation is considered only when heart failure reaches NYHA class IV or American College of Cardiology/American Heart Association (ACC/AHA) stage D. A patient is placed on the waiting list for a donor heart after careful evaluation to determine whether the treatment is appropriate and the patient is likely to survive the operation and regain normal function. There is no official cut-off age for transplantation, but the shortage of donor organs makes it unlikely that most older patients will receive an available heart.

Anyone being considered for a heart transplant must be willing to follow a strict diet, not smoke, and exercise regularly. They also must be capable of following a complex regimen of drugs to prevent the immune system from attacking the new organ. For patients who are deterred by the potential complications associated with lifelong immune-suppressant medications, or with other serious medical conditions, VADs may be a better option.

Perhaps more than any other operation, a transplant requires thoughtful consideration of psychological issues, because compliance with post-transplant medications, emotional stability, and a supportive environment of family and friends are critical to the long-term success of the new heart.

The name of every patient approved for transplantation is placed on the computerized UNOS list of people awaiting donor hearts. Seven tiers categorize patients from the most to least risk of dying.

- **Status 1 and 2** primarily include critically ill patients in the intensive care unit who have been placed on temporary, life-supporting mechanical circulatory support devices.
- **Status 3** primarily includes less critically ill patients who are being supported on intravenous medications or mechanical support devices. Some may be hospitalized; others are stable enough to be discharged.
- **Status 4, 5, and 6** includes patients who can be safely and comfortably maintained at home with intravenous or

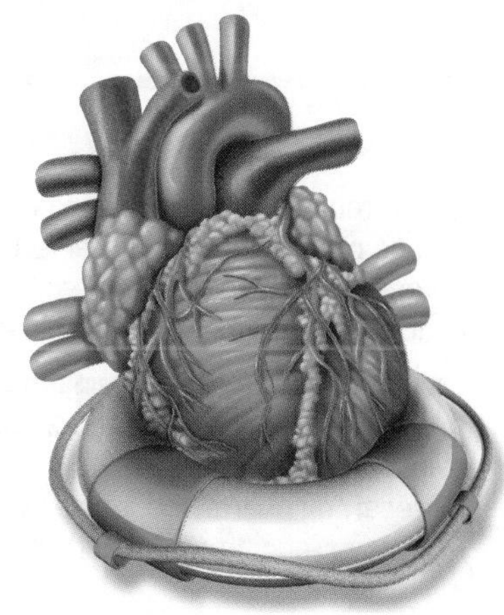

Heart transplantation is a lifesaver for heart failure patients who receive a donor heart—more than half of recipients survive for more than 12 years after the surgery.

More Patients Than Ever Receiving Heart Transplants

Heart transplants are available to selected patients with end-stage heart disease and no other serious medical issues. Patients are no longer automatically eliminated if they have human immunodeficiency virus (HIV), hepatitis C, low-grade cancer, or a number of other diseases.

Lack of donor organs remains the primary obstacle to receiving a new heart. In 2018, surgeons performed 3,408 heart transplants and 32 heart/lung transplants. As of August 1, 2019, 1,783 patients had received new hearts, with 23 receiving hearts and lungs. Yet there were 3,799 patients still waiting for a new heart, and 44 for a heart and lungs.

standard oral medications and/or stable mechanical support devices.

- **Status 7** includes patients who are temporarily unable to undergo a heart transplant.

UNOS follows carefully established rules on the allocation of organs. A few patients wait only days for a donor heart, while others wait months or years. The average wait in most parts of the United States is six to 12 months.

The Surgical Procedure. The transplant operation takes four to eight hours. Antirejection drugs are given before surgery while the patient is being prepared. During the operation, the patient is connected to a cardiopulmonary bypass (heart-lung) machine to take over the function of the heart and lungs. The diseased heart is removed as soon as the donor heart arrives in the operating room. The operation must be carefully coordinated to account for the time needed to pick up and deliver the donor heart, which may come from another part of the country.

Following the operation, patients are given intravenous medication, fluids, and drugs to prevent organ rejection. Remarkably, as early as the day after the transplant, patients may begin to eat and walk around. They are monitored in the hospital for one to three weeks before going home.

After Transplant Surgery. Heart transplant patients require lifelong medical care. Routine evaluations are necessary to gauge the new heart's performance and to monitor for rejection.

The biggest obstacle in heart transplantation is preventing the body from rejecting the donor heart. Powerful immunosuppressive drugs must be taken for life. These drugs can cause serious side effects, so their dosing must be carefully adjusted and monitored to get the maximum protection with the fewest side effects. Research is underway to find new and safer anti-rejection drugs.

Unfortunately, a transplanted heart is at increased risk of developing CAD due to a type of chronic rejection. Complications of post-transplant CAD are the most common cause of death after the first year. A drug called everolimus (Certican) showed promise in reducing this risk. It is widely used in Europe but has not been approved by the FDA for use in U.S. patients with CAD. However, it is approved for preventing organ rejection after kidney transplantation.

Transplantation is not the answer to the widespread problem of heart failure. No one expects that the supply of donor hearts will ever match the demand, and some patients are considered unsuitable candidates for transplantation. If you have been told you are inoperable due to a weak heart muscle, it may be wise to obtain a second opinion at a center specializing in heart failure and heart transplantation, such as Cleveland Clinic. High-risk bypass and valve operations are more often successfully performed at these centers. Some patients also are evaluated for a heart transplant before having high-risk surgery, so that a VAD can be used as a bridge to transplant or an alternative to transplantation if surgery does not improve the condition. Ask questions, do your research, and seek a second opinion if your doctor deems your condition to be serious and says that your options are limited.

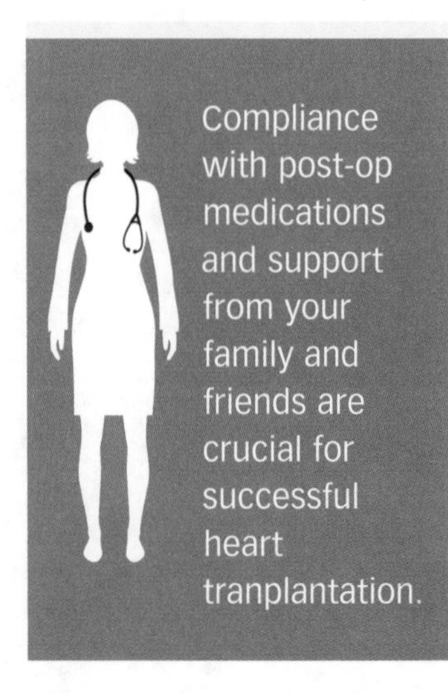

© Sharaf Maksumov | Dreamstime

Being diagnosed with heart failure is not the death sentence it once was.

9 Conclusion

Researchers are exploring many avenues in their efforts to uncover the secrets of heart failure and find better ways to improve the care of patients with this condition. Their goals include:

- Learning more about changes in cells that lead to heart failure
- Developing tests to detect the earliest signs of heart failure
- Identifying the factors that cause heart failure to worsen
- Researching new medical and surgical therapies
- Designing mechanical circulatory-assist devices
- Creating genetic tests to better determine who responds to heart failure medications
- Stopping damage from a heart attack to prevent heart failure
- Finding ways to reverse heart failure

Countless scientists and physicians are working diligently to find novel approaches to help slow the progression of heart failure, reverse it, and restore the damage it causes. Many clinical trials are being conducted at Cleveland Clinic on medications and devices for patients with heart failure. Researchers also are deciphering the genetics of heart failure. Exciting studies have produced evidence that the microbial composition of the digestive tract, as determined by diet, influences the prognosis in heart failure.

Tackling Diastolic Heart Failure

The medication and devices discussed in this report are primarily used in people who have heart failure with reduced ejection fraction (HFrEF), which also is known as systolic heart failure. In HFrEF, the heart's primary pumping chamber does not contract strongly enough to eject a sufficient amount of blood into the circulation. This causes the amount of blood ejected with each squeeze (ejection fraction) to drop.

As you read in Chapter 2, there is a second form of heart failure called heart failure with preserved ejection fraction (HFpEF), which also is known as diastolic heart failure. In HFpEF, the heart pumps well, but its walls are stiff and unable to expand properly. This prevents the heart from filling with blood at normal pressures. As a result, blood backs up in the lungs and circulation, causing shortness of breath and swelling. Medications to reduce these pressures and their associated symptoms have not been successful. As a result, people with HFpEF often require frequent hospitalizations for intravenous diuretic therapy. Due to the difficulty managing HFpEF, care by an experienced cardiologist is highly recommended.

The inter-atrial shunt device (IASD) was designed to tackle this problem. Now in clinical trials, it appears to do what drugs cannot. The IASD creates an opening between the right and left sides of the heart, so that blood can flow from the high-pressure left atrium to the low-pressure right atrium. This lowers the pressure in the left atrium and lungs. In the first IASD study, patients who received the device showed lasting improvements in New York Heart Association class and quality of life and were able to walk further without fatigue. Cleveland Clinic plans to participate in clinical trials of this device.

Much research is ongoing into the use of stem cells in heart failure treatment. Questions remain over what type of stem cells are most effective, how many should be used, and how they should be administered.

Cardiologist-Led Care Keeps Heart Failure Patients Out of the Hospital

Patients with diastolic heart failure admitted to the hospital under the care of a cardiologist are less likely to be rehospitalized within seven days of being discharged than those admitted by an internist. The reason appears to be that cardiologists are more comfortable prescribing aggressive diuretic therapy. A 2017 study of heart-failure patients admitted to a single tertiary care center over a four-month period found that those managed by a cardiologist also were more likely to be discharged with an outpatient cardiology appointment within seven days. Such continuity of care is known to be effective in reducing the rate of rehospitalization.

The study found that medically complex patients—those with pneumonia, diabetes, or pulmonary disease, for example—tended to be admitted under the care of an internist. Those with underlying cardiac problems, such as an arrhythmia or valve disease, were admitted by a cardiologist.

Where Stem Cell Research Stands

The potential to regenerate dysfunctional or lost heart muscle using stem cells is an intriguing area of research.

Stem cells are immature cells with the ability to become any kind of tissue, depending on where they are needed. The body releases about 30,000 stem cells into the bloodstream every day. Researchers are trying to harness the power of these versatile, multipurpose cells to repair damage from heart disease. Yet despite concerted efforts, stem-cell therapy is unlikely to become a viable treatment within the next few years.

Among the issues yet to be determined are the type of stem cell that works best, how they should be given to a patient, and how many cells are needed to produce effective results. Unfortunately, most of the clinical trials done to date have been too small to draw firm conclusions, and conclusions reached by similar trials often have been contradictory. Although a consensus often can be reached by combining the data from many clinical trials into large meta-analysis, there is too much variety in stem cell trials to take this approach: It would be like comparing apples and oranges.

Here's what we know so far about stem cell therapy:

- In the United States, you must be in a clinical trial to receive stem cell therapy.
- Bone marrow-derived mononuclear stem cells (BMMS) are safe and do not produce a reaction from the immune system that requires treatment with

immunosuppressant drugs.

- Mesenchymal stem cells (MSCs) also may be safe, but the jury is still out.
- Skeletal myoblasts are no longer used, because they cause potentially deadly arrhythmias.
- Stem cells that are taken from younger people are more robust than those taken from older individuals.
- Stem cells that are taken from the patient and returned to the patient (autogenic cells) are safe. Stem cells taken from another person (allogenic) also can be safely used, which gives older heart failure patients hope for a better outcome.
- Stem cells can be effective when delivered directly into the heart muscle or into a coronary artery.
- After being injected, stem cells may not take root and populate. Instead, they may release substances that recruit the host tissue to repair the damage. The stem cells themselves disappear after several weeks, but their beneficial effect may last as long as six months.
- When stem cells cause a measurable improvement in the heart—for example, by minimizing scar tissue, increasing blood flow to the heart muscle, or improving a heart failure patient's ejection fraction—heart function may not noticeably improve. When significant improvement in heart function does occur, it usually takes the form of improved ejection fraction.
- Large, well-designed studies that are now underway will increase our understanding of whether the effects of stem-cell therapy can decrease symptoms of heart failure and improve survival.

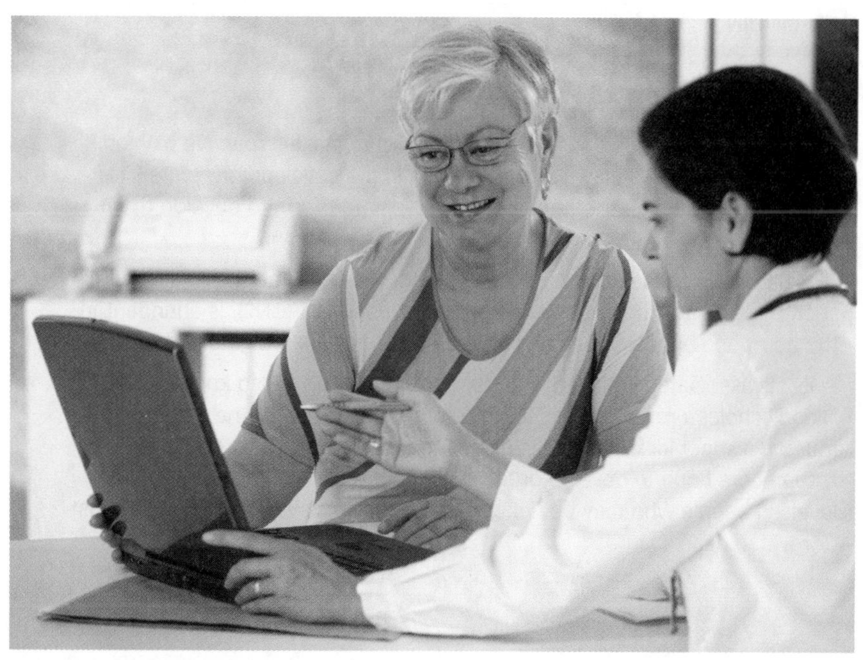

Work closely with your doctor to preserve your heart function.

Investigating the Role of Genes

Genes are now known to be responsible for heart failure in up to one-third of patients—perhaps more. Many of these patients have a form of cardiomyopathy that is genetically transmitted.

Cleveland Clinic cardiologists now offer genetic testing to heart failure patients when an underlying genetic cause for developing this condition is suspected. This usually involves individuals who have hypertrophic cardiomyopathy or familial cardiomyopathy (covered in Chapter 2). A positive genetic test also signals that the patient's siblings and children should be tested. If they also carry the gene, they will be able to take steps to prevent heart failure before it occurs.

Knowing which genes play a role in heart failure also provides researchers with novel therapeutic targets. One of these genes is SERCA2A, which helps heart cells maintain proper levels of calcium. Low SERCA2A levels adversely affect the heart's ability to contract. Cleveland Clinic has participated in the first human trial to test whether reintroducing the gene for SERCA2A into these patients can improve

NEW FINDING

Rallying the Body to Protect the Heart

Persistent inflammation and the generation of damaging reactive oxygen and nitrogen species play a significant role in the development of heart failure. Anti-oxidative treatments might help, but efforts to develop them have failed.

Cleveland Clinic researchers have identified a key enzyme that may lead to such treatments. The enzyme, called paraoxonase 2 (PON2), is abundant in the heart and appears to protect it against stress when it gets overexcited.

PON2 is associated with high-density lipoprotein (HDL), also known as "good" cholesterol). In studies of mice with heart disease, the researchers found a distinct lack of PON2 in damaged hearts. In the future, these researchers hope to develop drugs or other methods of improving PON2 levels in people who may be deficient, to raise HDL levels and guard against or reverse heart failure.

Free Radical Biology & Medicine, June 2018

the heart's pumping ability and reverse heart failure.

Genetic variants also are proving useful in determining the likelihood of a patient responding to some heart failure medications, such as beta-blockers, thereby taking the guesswork out of treatment. In the future, genetic tests may be used to eliminate trial and error by determining in advance which drug will work best for an individual.

Preventing Heart Failure

The ultimate goal is preventing heart failure from occurring—or at minimum, nipping it in the bud. Cleveland Clinic researchers have now identified an enzyme that protects the heart against reactive oxygen stress. They are optimistic that creating drugs to raise blood levels of this enzyme may guard against or reverse heart failure (see "Rallying the Body to Protect the Heart").

Remain Hopeful

The key message in this report is that heart failure is not always progressive and irreversible. Early treatment can slow progression of the condition. Although heart failure is a complex problem, take heart: By working closely with a heart failure specialist, you can be assured of receiving the latest and best treatments. This will enable you to live longer and enjoy a better quality of life.

If you have heart failure, you may hear many of the terms used in this report but not always understand what they mean. This glossary is designed to help you. If you want more information on any term, ask your doctor.

ablation: The destruction of heart tissue, usually with heat, cold, or sound waves. In patients with abnormal heart rhythms, ablation is sometimes used to destroy tissue that is causing the rhythm disturbance.

ambulatory monitors: Small portable electrocardiograph machines that record the heart's rhythm. Each type of monitor has unique features related to length of recording time and ability to send recordings over the phone. They include the Holter monitor, loop recorder, and transtelephonic transmitter. These monitors are used to measure changes in blood pressure throughout the day, and can be worn while going about everyday activities.

angina (also called angina pectoris): Discomfort or pain in the chest that occurs when fatty plaques that narrow coronary arteries interfere with blood supply to the heart muscle. Discomfort also may be felt in the neck, jaw, or arms. Stable angina usually occurs during periods of physical or emotional stress and is relieved by rest. Unstable angina can occur at any time, even during periods of rest or mild exertion.

angiotensin converting enzyme (ACE) inhibitors: Drugs that dilate blood vessels to improve the heart's output and increase blood flow to the kidneys. ACE inhibitors block the adverse effects of the hormone angiotensin II.

angiotensin receptor blockers (ARBs): Drugs that dilate blood vessels by blocking the effects of angiotensin II at the tissue level. They are similar to ACE inhibitors but have fewer side effects.

antiarrhythmics: Drugs that control the heart's rhythm.

anticoagulants: Drugs that prevent blood from clotting.

aorta: The large, main artery exiting the heart. All blood pumped out of the left ventricle travels through the aorta on its way to other parts of the body.

arrhythmias: Abnormal heart rhythms.

atherosclerosis: Hardening or narrowing of the arteries due to deposits of fatty substances, cholesterol, calcium, and fibrin (the protein that forms a blood clot) that slow or block blood flow.

atrial fibrillation: A heart-rhythm disorder (arrhythmia) in which the upper chambers of the heart (atria) contract rapidly, creating a fast, irregular heart rhythm.

beta-blockers: Drugs that modulate the activity of the sympathetic nervous system, slowing the heart rate and reducing blood pressure. In patients with heart failure, beta-blockers improve survival, slow the progression of heart failure, improve New York Heart Association functional class, and reduce the risk of hospitalization. They also may prevent ventricular remodeling and arrhythmias.

blood clot (thrombus): A clot forms when clotting factors in the blood cause it to coagulate or become a jelly-like mass. When a blood clot forms inside a blood vessel, it can dislodge, travel through the bloodstream, and become trapped, causing a heart attack or stroke.

bradycardia: A slow heart rate.

bypass: A surgical procedure designed to increase blood flow to an organ or extremity by rerouting blood around a blocked artery.

cachexia: Drastic loss of weight, muscle, and bone throughout the body.

calcification: A process in which tissue becomes hardened due to deposits of calcium salts. Calcification of blood vessels plays a role in the development of atherosclerosis.

calcium-channel blocker: A drug that reduces blood vessel spasms, lowers blood pressure, and controls angina.

cardiac catheterization: An imaging procedure that involves inserting a catheter into a blood vessel in the arm or leg and guiding it to the heart with the aid of x-ray movies. Contrast dye injected through the catheter allows the coronary arteries to be seen (coronary angiography).

cardiac output: The amount of blood the heart pumps out in one minute, measured in liters per minute.

cardiomyopathies: A group of diseases that primarily affect the heart muscle.

clinical trials: Research studies that test medical treatments in humans. The optimal clinical trials are randomized, placebo-controlled studies, meaning the participants are randomly assigned to treatment groups, and one group receives a placebo (inactive pill or device) and the other receives the study drug or device. In double-blind trials, neither the researchers nor the patients know which therapy any patient has received until the study is over. This removes any chance of bias in the results.

congestion: Excess fluid in the tissues and organs.

coronary artery disease (CAD): A build-up of fatty material in the walls of the coronary artery (atherosclerosis) that narrows the artery.

cyanosis: Blue lips and fingernails caused by inadequate oxygenated blood in the extremities.

decompensation: A sudden increase in symptoms such as difficulty breathing, indicating the heart is no longer able to pump with enough force to keep blood circulating properly. Decompensated heart failure requires immediate hospitalization for intravenous diuretics.

deep vein thrombosis (DVT): A clot in a deep vein, usually in the leg. Symptoms may include pain and swelling, but there may be no symptoms at all. If untreated, the clot may travel to the lungs, where it can cause a fatal pulmonary embolism.

diabetes: A disease that affects the body's ability to metabolize sugar, either because the pancreas does not produce insulin (type 1 diabetes), a hormone that regulates the absorption of sugar from the bloodstream, or because the body is resistant to the effects of insulin (type 2 diabetes).

diastolic pressure: The blood pressure in the arteries when the heart is filling with blood. It is the lower of two blood pressure measurements—for example, in a blood pressure reading of 120/80 millimeters of mercury (mmHg), 80 is the diastolic pressure.

digoxin: A drug that increases the heart's pumping ability.

diuretics: Drugs that remove excess fluid from the tissues and bloodstream, lessen edema (swelling), and make breathing easier. These are sometimes called water pills.

dyspnea: Shortness of breath.

echocardiogram (ECG): An imaging procedure that creates a moving picture of the heart's valves and chambers using high-frequency sound waves emanating from a device placed on the chest or guided into the esophagus behind the heart. Echocardiography is used to evaluate blood flow through the heart's valves.

edema: Swelling from water retention.

ejection fraction: The percentage of blood in the ventricles pumped out with each beat. A normal ejection fraction is 55 to 65 percent. The lower the percentage, the more advanced the heart failure.

exercise stress test: A test used to provide information about how the heart responds to stress. It usually involves walking on a treadmill or pedaling a stationary bike at increasing levels of difficulty, while your heart rate and blood pressure are monitored. Alternatively, medications may be used to simulate the effect of exercise on the heart.

heart failure (congestive heart failure, CHF): A chronic, progressive disease in which the heart muscle weakens and no longer can pump blood well enough to meet the body's needs.

hemodynamic: Pertaining to pressures and movements in the circulation of blood.

hibernating myocardium: Heart muscle cells that appear dead after a heart attack but revive after blood flow is restored.

hypertension: High blood pressure.

hyperkalemia: Elevated potassium levels.

hypertrophy: An abnormal enlargement of an organ or thickening of its tissue.

idiopathic: Of unknown cause.

inotropic agent: A type of drug that stimulates the heart to contract.

ischemia: Inadequate blood supply to the heart muscle (or any other organ or tissue).

left ventricular assist device (LVAD): An implanted mechanical device that pumps blood directly to assist a failing heart.

myocardial perfusion: A measure of how the heart muscle is nourished by blood.

myocardium: The heart muscle.

neurohormonal: Of both the neural (nervous) and hormonal (hormone) systems.

pacemaker: An electronic device that is implanted under the skin and sends electrical impulses to the heart muscle to maintain a desired heart rate.

pericardium: The sac that surrounds the heart.

pulse rate: The number of heartbeats per minute. The resting pulse rate for an average adult is between 60 and 100 beats per minute (BPM).

orthopnea: Shortness of breath that occurs when lying down.

paroxysmal nocturnal dyspnea: Awakening from sleep at night with shortness of breath.

rales: Crackling noises in the lungs that can be heard with a stethoscope.

remodeling: Changes in the size, shape, and function of the heart and its blood vessels.

revascularization: Procedures, such as coronary artery bypass grafting and balloon angioplasty with stenting, that restore or increase blood flow through a coronary artery.

septum: The wall between the two ventricles.

stroke volume: The amount of blood pumped out each time the heart contracts.

systolic pressure: The pressure of the blood in the arteries when the heart contracts. It is the higher of two blood pressure measurements—for example, in a blood pressure reading of 120/80 mmHg, 120 is the systolic pressure.

vasodilators: Drugs that cause blood vessels to relax, improving blood flow.

ventricular fibrillation: An abnormal heart rhythm that is similar to atrial fibrillation but causes the ventricles (the lower chambers of the heart) to quiver in a rapid and uncoordinated way. Without immediate treatment to stabilize the heart rate, cardiac arrest and death may occur.

ventricular tachycardia: An abnormal heart rhythm characterized by a heart rate of 100 beats per minute or more, combined with three or more irregular beats in a row. Ventricular tachycardia can be a medical emergency, and can develop into ventricular fibrillation if untreated.

Cleveland Clinic Heart and Vascular Institute
www.myclevelandclinic.org/departments/heart
800-659-7822
9500 Euclid Ave.
Cleveland, OH 44195

American Heart Association National Center
www.heart.org
800-242-8721
7272 Greenville Ave.
Dallas, TX 75231

National Heart, Lung and Blood Institute
www.nhlbi.nih.gov
301-496-4000
NHLBI Health Information Center
Building 31
31 Center Dr.
Bethesda, MD 20892

American College of Cardiology
www.acc.org
resource@acc.org
800-253-4636, ext. 5603
2400 N. Street NW
Washington, DC 20037

Heart Failure Society of America
www.hfsa.org
info@hfsa.org
301-312-8635
9211 Corporate Blvd., Suite 270
Rockville, MD 20850

American Society of Transplantation
www.myast.org
856-439-9986
1120 Rte. 73, Suite 200
Mt. Laurel, NJ 08054

If you're experiencing any of these symptoms:

CALL YOUR DOCTOR

- Weight gain of more than three pounds in one day or five pounds in one week
- Swelling in your ankles, legs, or abdomen that has become worse
- Shortness of breath that has become worse, especially if you awaken short of breath
- Extreme fatigue or decreased activity tolerance
- A respiratory infection or cough that has become worse
- Fast heart rate (100 beats per minute or more)
- Episodes of chest pain or discomfort with exertion that are relieved with rest
- Difficulty breathing with normal activities or at rest
- Severe dizziness, lightheadedness, or fainting
- Nausea or poor appetite

CALL 911

Call 911 if you are experiencing any of the symptoms of a heart attack:

- New chest pain or discomfort that is severe, unexpected, and accompanied by shortness of breath, sweating, nausea, or weakness, and/or is unrelieved by nitroglycerin
- Fast, sustained heart rate (more than 120 beats per minute), especially if you are short of breath, dizzy, or lightheaded
- Shortness of breath that is not relieved by rest
- Sudden weakness or paralysis in your arms or legs
- Loss of consciousness

IN CASE OF EMERGENCY

Fill in these details and leave them in a prominent place (for example, taped to the refrigerator) for family, friends, and paramedics in case of emergency.

MY DATE OF BIRTH AND AGE:

MY ADDRESS:

MY PHONE NUMBER:

MY INSURANCE INFORMATION:

MY DOCTOR'S NAME AND ADDRESS:

MY DOCTOR'S PHONE NUMBER:

NAME AND ADDRESS OF HOSPITAL, NEAREST TO ME:

MY PHARMACY (NAME, PHONE, ADDRESS):

MY MEDICATIONS (INCLUDE DOSAGE):

Use this form if you are recovering from heart failure at home

Fluid Measurements

1 ounce = 30 mL

8 ounces = 240 mL

1 cup = 8 ounces = 240 mL

Sample Measurements

Coffee cup = 200 mL

Small milk carton = 240 mL

Juice, Jello, or ice cream cup = 120 mL

Soup bowl = 160 mL

Your daily fluid limit is ____________

Your daily sodium limit is ____________

FLUID INTAKE

6 a.m. to 2 p.m.

Type of Fluid	Amount
____________	______ mL
____________	______ mL
____________	______ mL
____________	______ mL
____________	______ mL
Total	______ mL

2 p.m. to 10 p.m.

Type of Fluid	Amount
____________	______ mL
____________	______ mL
____________	______ mL
____________	______ mL
____________	______ mL
Total	______ mL

10 p.m. to 6 a.m.

Type of Fluid	Amount
____________	______ mL
____________	______ mL
____________	______ mL
Total	______ mL

Daily Total ____________ mL

SODIUM INTAKE

6 a.m. to 2 p.m.

Amount

____________ mg
____________ mg
____________ mg
____________ mg
____________ mg
Total ____________ mg

2 p.m. to 10 p.m.

Amount

____________ mg
____________ mg
____________ mg
____________ mg
____________ mg
Total ____________ mg

10 p.m. to 6 a.m.

Amount

____________ mg
____________ mg
____________ mg
Total ____________ mg

Daily Total ____________ mg

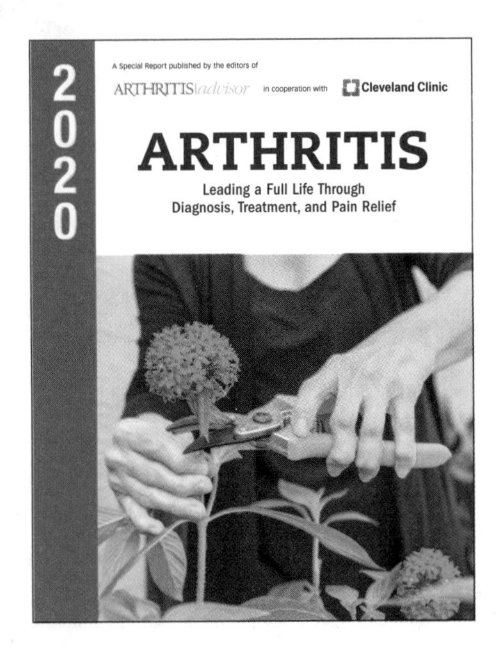

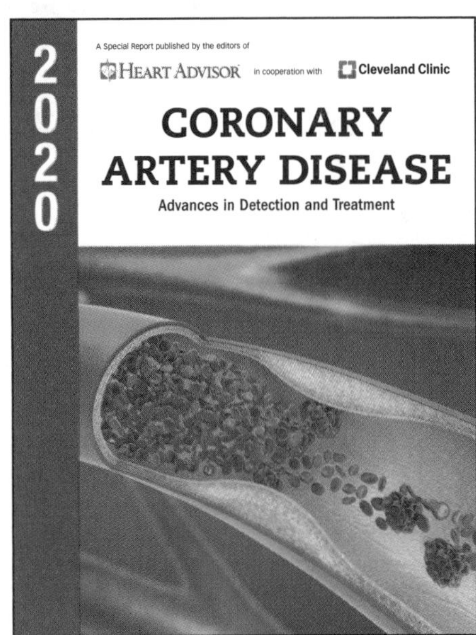

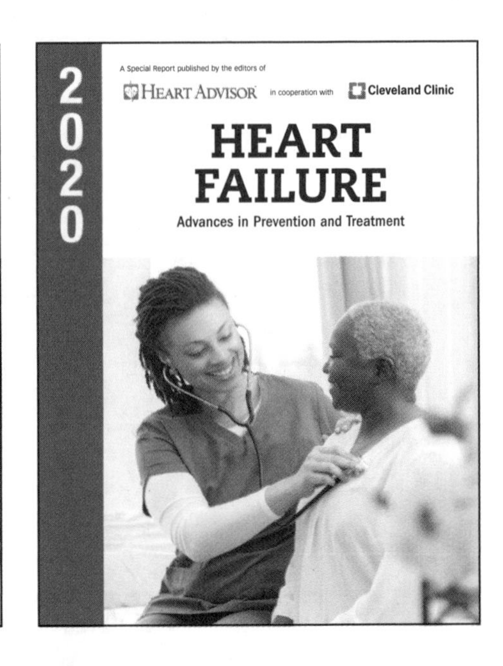

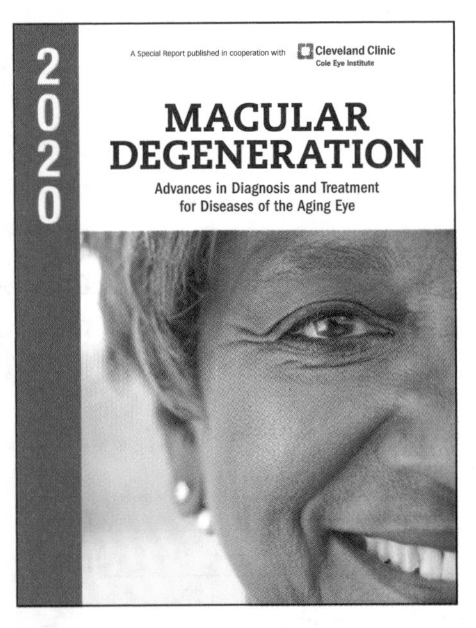

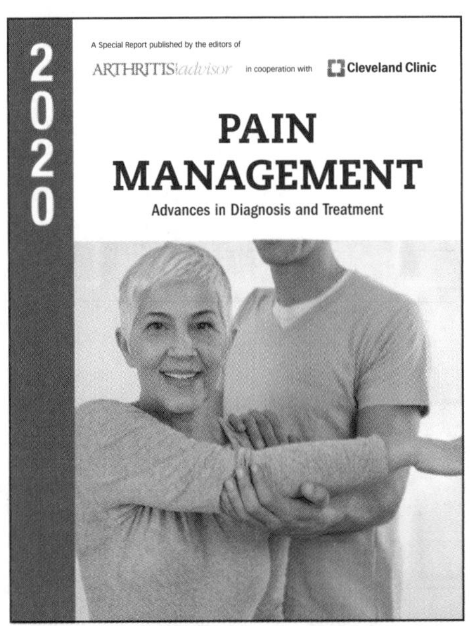

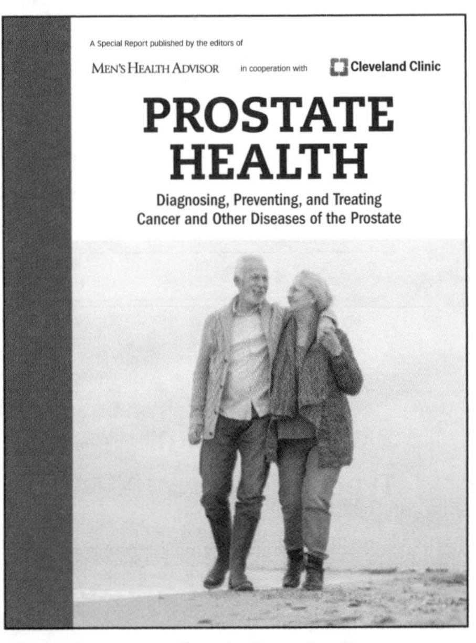

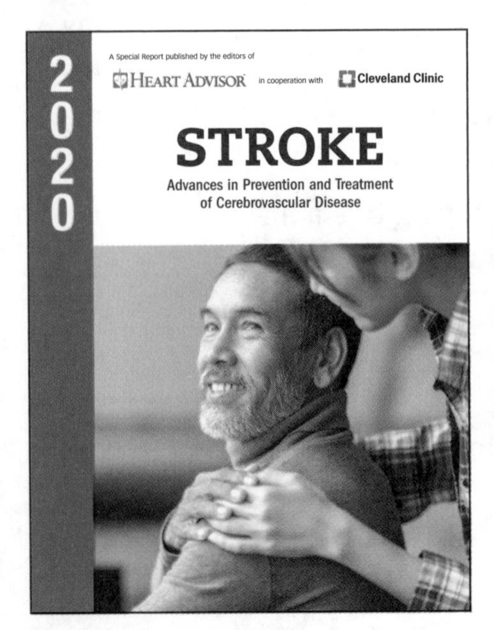

2020 HEALTH SPECIAL REPORTS

ORDER NOW

For print copies of health reports,
call 877-300-0253.

For digital or print copies, go to:
heart-advisor.com/subscribe